Tapping Feet

A Double-take on Care Homes and Dementia

by

Lewine Mair

Text © Lewine Mair, 2022
All rights reserved.
Typeset in 12pt Times New Roman

Most characters and events in this publication, other than those clearly in the public domain, are fictitious, but some are based on the fine collection of people I have met, with all names changed and some events modified for the story.

Cover Photo Image Credit: Dmitry Zyrin – iStock.com

Head for Change.
Be part of the solution

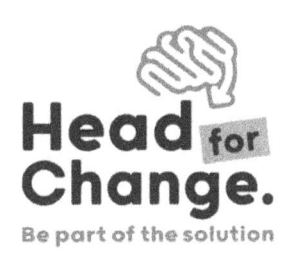

Head for Change is a recently-formed charitable foundation, pioneering positive change for brain health in sport and supporting ex-players who are affected by neurodegenerative disease as a result of their professional sporting career in football or rugby. In addition, they work with researchers internationally, as well as providing educational opportunities for players and the wider footballing community, to inform on the dangers of sports-related injuries. Their core mission is 'to be part of the solution'.

Head for Change, the book's charitable partner, will receive 32.5% of the profit from each sale of Tapping Feet.

Acknowledgements

To my family, who encouraged me to go ahead with a book which was for long nothing more than a diary scribbled in the years when my husband had dementia. There came a day when Venetia, the fourth among my seven grandchildren, asked if she could read a couple of pages. I plucked up the courage to let her have a look, and it was her reaction which gave me the courage I needed to continue.

Next, the oldest granddaughter, Jenni, looked through the chapters with a doctor's eye and found the book a good read in the process. My thanks to both of them and to my sons and daughters, Logan, Patrick, Suzi and Michele, who were no different from the grandchildren in scrutinising the contents and contributing plenty of their own memories. "Get on with it!" was their most oft-repeated message.

Jenni's younger sisters, Victoria and the twins, Jessica and Charlotte, added to the whole with their penchant for doing daily "ward rounds" at Norman's care home when they got off the bus from school. As Connie, the matron, said recently, "They didn't just visit Norman, they visited everyone." As for Olivia and Alex, Venetia's sister and brother, and Logan's wife, Rachel, and her father, Charles Woodhouse, they too, liked the odd progress report, with Rachel contributing a welcome last-minute read.

My sister Miranda, a retired social worker, and some of her social-work friends, were never less than helpful, as was Patricia Davies, a work colleague with whom I have this excellent relationship: neither of us is afraid to tell the other what she thinks.

Finally, my thanks to Ron Black from Lindemann Health Care and his staff for advice on care homes in general, and to Garry Pierrepont and Tony Davies, who liked my approach to our family's experience of the dementia situation enough to take on the editing and self-publishing side of the process. Add in the knowledge brought to bear by Lorna Fergusson, my coach on a creative writing course at Oxford, and my daughter, Michele, a PR Executive in the Golf Department of IMG, and *Tapping Feet, a Double-take on Care Homes and Dementia* turned into the book we have here.

Contents

Introduction

Chapter 1: Disconcerting Days 2007-2012

Chapter 2: Decisions

Chapter 3: Farrow Hall

Chapter 4: A Wimbledon Final to Remember

Chapter 5: Advantage Alicia

Chapter 6: A Lesson

Chapter 7: A Mixed Club

Chapter 8: Moments

Chapter 9: Save the Last Dance for me

Chapter 10: Lost and Found

Chapter 11: The Great Escape

Chapter 12: Hang On to What You've Got

Chapter 13: Yellow Dusters

Chapter 14: Puzzling

Chapter 15: The Christmas Party

Chapter 16: Who is Wearing What

Chapter 17: The Other Half

Chapter 18: A Bridge Too Far

Chapter 19: The Last Laugh

Chapter 20: A Taste of Trouble

Chapter 21: Warning Strokes

Chapter 22: Short Shrift from Nakita

Postscript

Lewine Mair

Tapping Feet

A Double-take on Care Homes and Dementia

Introduction

There was a touch of magic about the new piano I had volunteered to play at the care home where my then 84-year-old husband was a resident for the last two-and-a-half years of his eight-year fight with dementia. After I had completed the first half of 'On the Street where you Live' from *My Fair Lady*, it almost took off on its own, moving seamlessly into that old Cole Porter number, 'Anything Goes'.

And that is when I noticed a bit more magic.

At least ten of the men and women sitting in the room were tapping their feet, with some among the hardest hit of the dementia patients appearing to be as taken with the music as the other residents. Instead of staring absentmindedly at whatever was or was not happening in front of them, they had burst into life like characters in a musical box. The pattern was no different the next time I played and the next and, before too long, these musical interludes started to inspire some of the stories in this book. Time and time again, an old tune would be at the heart of the tale: the story of Betsy and her doting husband, Henry, who visited her on a daily basis, is a case in point. Buoyed by the music, the two of them danced their way back into a happier past in which they had spent much of their retirement dancing around the world.

In the chapters that follow, I have used the name Farrow Hall – this came into my head after I purchased a sample pot of Farrow & Ball paint – to encompass Norman's care home and the four other sincerely good establishments which feature in these pages.

All are sited in Edinburgh or between Edinburgh and Livingston.

The scene-setting early chapters, along with those at the finish, tell of my husband's dementia journey after blissful years of playing rugby and writing on sport. Officially, he had a mix of dementia and Alzheimer's but, with the symptoms largely the same, I have simplified things by referring to the twin conditions as 'dementia'.

Sundry textbooks have been written on the subject and, in the medical sense, they tell you everything you need to know. But the problem I had with them was that they often made for relentlessly grim reading.

In Norman's case, we never knew what to expect next. There were plenty of the darker days, but every now and then there was the odd shaft of light and laughter which helped to balance the ledger.

Political correctness does not come naturally to your usual dementia victim and the residents at Farrow Hall were not immune from delivering their share of inappropriate comments. Of course, some of the newer residents' visitors would look appalled at what they were hearing, but it was seldom too long before what they might once have seen as an offensive comment would prompt a wry smile. For example, it was impossible not to enjoy that exchange between a nonagenarian lady by name of Hilda, and Norman, after she had alerted Norman to the fact that he had his sweater on back-to-front. His riposte to this classy and ancient aristocrat was an outrageous, "You're not looking so hot yourself."

As applies with all the care homes under the Farrow Hall label, I have disguised the names of residents and staff members alike, sometimes creating hybrid characters by way of keeping identities further under wraps in the various tales which are in the heart of this book. (If sometimes only loosely, all of these stories are based on truth.) Norman's name is one which remains unchanged, with the explanation, here, that I wanted to encourage people to talk about dementia rather than lock it inside the walls of a care home.

Not everyone will agree, but it has to be good news that rugby players and footballers are playing their part in the process by finally speaking out about the damage posed by head injuries in their sports and what can lie in store. Though Norman was a rugby player who played for Melrose and for Scotland before being admitted to Scottish Rugby's Hall of Fame in his later years, they did not worry about such things in his day.

He was lucky insofar as he died well before the advent of Covid-19. But for those who have coincided with the Covid years, there is no question that their care-home experiences have been very different. It takes all three of patients, visitors and a good team of care workers to create the sense of community on which these places thrive and, in the past few years, the above components have not always come together. Staff have had to isolate at home; residents have at times been deprived of visitors and, still worse, they have had to be confined to their own rooms. In the programme *Inside the Care Crisis with Ed Balls*, which was aired at the start of 2022, the politician revealed that one in four care homes in England was on the brink of financial collapse. The managers of these establishments could not afford to pay the care-home workers what they felt they should be paying them, while their own expenses had shot up because of the changes – often to do with equipment – which had come into play during the Covid years.

Yet things can only get better for care homes and residents alike, and my hope is that this book will serve as a reminder that there can be plenty of spirited interaction in a care home, just as there is anywhere else.

As you read the following pages, I'll introduce you to a range of characters who might touch your heart and maybe entertain you, while all the time serving as reminders of our common humanity.

Chapter 1: Disconcerting Days 2007-2012

No one wants to believe what they are seeing when the early signs of dementia start to manifest themselves. Where someone does something to suggest that things are not quite right, even family members (and in Norman's case that included me during the initial stages) can be inclined to make excuses on the person's behalf. They will suggest that the latest aberration is nothing to worry about; old Mrs So-and-So from up the road was wearing a new outfit, so no wonder she was not easily recognisable. To pretend that nothing is happening is just one way of dealing with the subject. For another, one which was used by several of our acquaintances, an enquiry into the victim's health is apt to be followed by a hasty switch of subject. You don't want to regale anyone with information they would prefer not to hear, but at times it can make a wife/husband/partner feel no less hopelessly isolated than the victim.

When less nervous folk were moved to question Norman about what he was doing or saying, they would often find themselves on the end of a sharp put-down. For instance, when Doctor Smyth, then his GP, eventually coaxed him into taking a cognitive assessment, he issued a stern rebuke. As far as he was concerned, the questions he was being asked were so asinine as to suggest that the doctor should be worried about his own state of health.

Dr Smyth would explain to me later that, in his experience at least, dementia sufferers tended to go one of two ways. They could become acquiescent or they could become angry, and often wily with it. Norman, who had been breathtakingly perceptive in so many areas in his days as writer, fell into the second category. His coping mechanism, for most of the eight years over which his condition developed, was to view what was happening to him as someone else's fault. And if it was not the doctor's fault, it was mine.

It was about four years into his decline that I became acutely aware that he needed to stop driving. There had been a series of bumps and close calls, none of which, apparently, was down to him. He would point out that his record as a driver was unblemished and even said as much to the poor fellow who accused him of cannoning into his shiny white van. Norman, who had studied law at university years before, left the poor chap wishing he had never mentioned it.

I tried to call a halt to such scenes by driving him everywhere. Sometimes it worked but, virtually every day, he would be adamant that he wished to go here or there on his own. You will be thinking that the answer was ridiculously simple. Hide the keys. I did that on multiple occasions, but the usual outcome was an angry rerun of his obsessive notion that I had stolen the car.

Even now, I have hair-raising memories of the day he happened upon the keys and went shooting up the road with a lurch and a roar.

I resorted to my old habit of chewing fingernails until he drew up outside the house at least two hours and half-a-tank of petrol later. You could sense that he, too, was shaken as he admitted to having got "a little lost" on his way to a nearby golf range. "A little lost", as the family would discover, involved a seventy-mile round trip to Melrose in the Scottish Borders, a town for whom he had played rugby years earlier.

The doctor made a gallant effort to get across a "no driving" message which, strictly speaking, was not for him to deliver. And when he was no more successful than the family had been in making it stick, he recommended that we call on the services of experts in the Mental Health Department at the local hospital. They would know how to get the job done.

In the knowledge that Norman would refuse to enter a door labelled "Mental Health Department" (this was how it read then, if not now) the doctor arranged a home visit.

The expert who came to call had been well-primed by Dr Smyth as to what kind of reception she might expect. She talked to Norman on her own for ten minutes before flying into the kitchen to deliver her thoughts to my daughter, Michele, and me, rather than to her patient. "Given that giving up driving is something he'll never agree to do," she said, "I think it would be easier to sell the car."

"Easier for whom?" I muttered under my breath.

There was shopping to be done and there were grandchildren to be collected from school. Also, Norman needed to be taken out as opposed to sitting in the house morning and afternoon. How was all that going to work?

I had a colleague called Kim who had been experiencing a similar set of problems with her father, a man who had grown progressively more impossible with the passing years. He had scoffed at his daughter's recommendation that he might do better to stop driving but, in an unfortunate event which doubled as a stroke of good fortune thanks to the inadequacy of the DVLA rules, the right thing happened at the right time. The old man reversed his car into someone's Ford Fiesta at the bowling club, rather than into what he thought was an empty space. The Fiesta's astonished owner was looking on. In the wake of that incident, the culprit went straight round to his daughter's house and hurled the car keys across the room. After that, to all-round relief, he moved on to a stage in the dementia process when he was only interested in pottering round the garden.

The different steps are more than passing strange. In Norman's case, his insistence on being allowed to drive gave way to a period in which he could no longer work the remote control gadget for the TV, whilst refusing to let anyone else touch it. This coincided with a stretch when he would open the washing machine in mid-cycle and the water would pour out on to the kitchen floor tiles. The tiles have never stayed bedded down since. These problems, in turn, led to a phase where he insisted on stepping into the bath rather than the shower and, on two occasions, the fire-brigade had to be called to help him get out. They said that they it was not something they could keep doing. Next on a fast-developing list was his wish to be taken to "the other house": a house we did not have.

Since there were times when he could not be dissuaded, I would play along with the idea in the faint hope that the trip might not be so crazy after all. Perhaps it would lead to one of several houses where he had lived in his youth.

The first of those outings began with my apparently turning the wrong way at the top of the road. I was to head instead towards the airport.

That instruction was clear enough, as was his conversation on the way, containing as it did some memories of his once-regular trips to Dublin in his capacity as a rugby writer. (Judging from recent research, it has seemed ever more likely that the fact that Norman had played rugby himself for many more years than most could well have contributed to his mental decline.)

When, on the day in question, we reached the road leading to the airport and I asked, "Where next?", he issued a further assortment of instructions, each of them making less sense than its predecessor. Ten minutes later, when we came face to face with a 'No Through Road' sign, I suggested we head instead for his favourite coffee shop.

The "second home" forgotten, we enjoyed a coffee and went home. Relatively speaking, the morning had been a triumph, at least insofar as it had kept him occupied.

As the months progressed, the day-to-day misadventures became alarm bells, with Norman getting up and dressed three or four times in the night and calling for anything from his golf clubs to his gun. (He owned golf clubs but not the gun.) Trying to persuade him to get undressed and go back to bed became the proverbial nightmare. By day, he slept for some of the time and created havoc the rest, often turning on the oven and all the knobs on the cooker. This departure was sorted out by a local electrician who came along with a device which meant that nothing could stay on for longer than half an hour unless a tucked-away button had been pressed.

Michele came up for a week at the start of November 2011 and insisted that I spend two or three nights in a local hotel in order to get a bit of sleep.

A nearby Travelodge was my hostelry of choice on the grounds that anything else would have felt wickedly self-indulgent. It worked well enough for me, but Michele, though she did not let me know quite how bad things were at the time, had the golf-club and the gun routine more often than I had ever done. That apart, Norman seemed to think she was in charge of a 24-hour room service operation. At one point, when she went down to the shops to get the newspapers he said he had to read over breakfast, he took it upon himself to cook a boiled egg in a saucepan of fresh orange juice. The result was not good, with the egg and the saucepan blackened by the time Michele came back through the door. The other half of the packet of fresh orange juice had been decanted into the cat's bowl.

When a pale-faced Michele left to return to London, Norman was around to see her off. "Have you enjoyed your holiday?" he asked.

After three or four crazy nights back at home, I paid for the services of a private care organisation which came highly priced and, though I struggle to understand how, highly recommended. The contract read that an experienced carer (for experienced read 'a complete novice') would arrive at 10pm and leave at seven on the dot. The "leaving" part of it was accompanied by a list of rules, these including a price list corresponding to the number of minutes which passed after the deadline had been reached.

I returned to the Travelodge which, this time around, was not offering quite the same peaceful scenario in that there was a problem with one of the petrol pumps in the front yard. At regular intervals through the night, there was a loudspeaker announcement to advise that "Pump Number 8", as I remember it so well, was out of order. On top of that, there was the unimaginable strain of that early-morning deadline. I defy anyone to get a half-decent night's sleep in such circumstances.

As it transpired, the situation had been just as bad back home. The novice care worker had been led a merry dance and, when Norman was up and dressed at two in the morning, she had left him sitting in a rocking chair watching television. In due course, the chair toppled over and Norman slipped to the floor. The girl did the right thing in covering him with his duvet but it was a moot point as to which of us, the care worker, Norman or myself, looked the worst for wear in the morning.

On another occasion, I went to sleep at Suzi's house (Suzi is the older of my two daughters and the mother of four daughters, Jenni, Victoria, and twins, Charlotte and Jessica). Suzi and Charlotte, in turn, came to our place.

Suzi was strict with regard to Norman's off-the-wall requests and, probably as a result, had no more than a couple of incidents. At three in the morning, he went to Charlotte's room to wake her up and tell her that she should be getting ready to play tennis. And a little later, it was about what Suzi would be giving him for breakfast. I, meantime, spent a comfortable night in Charlotte's bed, switching between sleep and looking at the stars.

Yet every now and then, there would be a better day, one when I would tell myself that things were not as bad as they seemed. Perhaps I was overreacting. Christmas Day worked surprisingly well, with Norman sitting quietly at the table while listening to the grandchildren's happy chatter and attempting to pull a few crackers. He even went down the garden for a few minutes to watch one of the twins hitting against the tennis club wall. New Year's Eve was another to pass without incident. When I made a hurried a trip to the hairdressers, he noticed as much on my return, even if his nasty little quip – "I hope it was painful" – was some way removed from the merriest of compliments. Patrick, the younger of my two sons, came round in the evening to do the night-time shift and, with Norman having gone to bed – and to sleep – at nine o'clock, we took advantage of this happy situation to watch a bit of TV before getting some sleep ourselves. Mercifully, there were no disturbances until, some time after midnight, the peace was interrupted by a spate of loud rings of the front-door bell. "Don't answer it," yelled my son, when he heard me heading downstairs.

The moment he joined me in the hall, the ringing stopped. Whoever it was – some drunkard we supposed, had moved on. Only then did we hear a voice. Norman's voice.

Though we never did discover when it was that he left the house, the rest of the story came out the next day. A resident from a couple of streets away had noticed him standing at the edge of the main road some half a mile from home and, on the assumption that he had been visiting friends, had offered to take him wherever he was going next. The moment it became clear that there was no rhyme or reason as to where that was, the said gentleman delivered him to our front door. His understandable conclusion was that his passenger had been drinking.

Norman was positively hyper when we let him in, and it was presumably because of it that he had been able to walk as far as he had when he was suffering from the beginnings of osteomyelitis, along with some other as yet undiagnosed problems. Only two nights earlier, it had taken a couple of the grandchildren – twins Charlotte and Jessica – to haul him up the stairs after he collapsed at the halfway point.

A friend, a medical man who lives just up the road, had warned there would be a crisis at some point and the crisis had come. For Norman, it was that appearance on a main road when no one was aware that he had left his bed. Dr Smyth, who had learned of events over the bush telegraph, came round on the morning after the walkabout and described the situation as "out of hand." Either Norman should be in a home or care workers should be coming to us. At the same time, he warned that nothing could happen in too much of a hurry. If we failed to go through the usual social work channels, we would not qualify for the grants which were on offer. Good thinking, only the social work department had more or less signed off for their Christmas and New Year break.

A series of ever-more frantic calls to the social work department resulted in the student manning the phone over the holiday period finally relenting as far as a consultation was concerned. He pencilled me in for what he termed "an emergency appointment".

Alas, my idea of an emergency appointment and his did not tally. The date on offer was three weeks away.

Chapter 2: Decisions

Doctor Smyth intervened and decided that the best way round the situation was for me to ask a nearby care home if they could take Norman for a fortnight in order to give the family a bit of respite. Farrow Hall was the nearest establishment, only that was not going to be ready until March at the earliest. However, the owner, John Marquis, a well-known horticulturist who was apparently related to the Duke of Littlestone, said that they had a small room available at one of his sister homes, The Stables, as from 8 January. First, though, the matron would need to come to the house to assess the prospective patient.

When she came, on 5 January, Norman confused her with one of his six sisters. He spoke to her agreeably enough, whilst at the same time claiming that he was in the best of health. The matron had been told about his osteomyelitis and, though he did admit to having had problems with his feet, he put them down to recent rugby and football injuries. The matron went along with his diagnosis.

Norman passed the test and, as I showed her out, she asked me to bring him along at 3 o'clock on the 8th.

In the knowledge that the handover would not be easy, I asked if we could link the arrangement to some foot treatment we had arranged for him that same afternoon. It was deceitful but it would be impossible to tell him the whole truth.

My sister Miranda, a former medical social worker who had often helped with Norman when I still had a busy work-schedule in my job as a part-time sportswriter, agreed to lend support.

Though a couple of ladies in wheelchairs was hardly what the two of us wanted to see as we approached the home's front door, a lively family group in the hallway lifted the mood, as did the sight of a pot of tea and a handsome Victoria Sponge on a side-room table.

Norman was still tucking into the cake when the matron summoned a nurse who was to join her in examining Norman's feet. The examination was about to start when the matron took one look at the latest bout of swelling and said that he would need to stay put for a few days to allow the staff to keep his feet in a raised position and get to the bottom of what was obviously a long-term problem. Norman went back to talking about sports' injuries and, as he passed on his thoughts to the nurse, so the matron recommended that Miranda and I should leave. She saw us to the door and advised that no one should visit that night for fear it might prove disruptive.

When I explained that Victoria, one of the grandchildren, had already made plans to turn up, the matron asked if I could put her off, just for that day. I sent the child a text.

Miranda and I fetched the overnight bag we had packed for Norman from the boot of the car and handed it in at reception. Then we disappeared. My heart was pounding, as much as it had at any time throughout those years of disrupted days and nights.

As my text to Victoria never arrived, she went ahead with her visit and turned up at the home as Norman was engaging in something known as the 'social hour' ahead of supper. He was talking to two ladies about hockey and Victoria joined in with the chat after he had introduced her with a surprising degree of accuracy. "This is Victoria," he began. "Her hockey team is unbeaten and she is the captain."

The hockey chat over, he moved on to talk about camps and soldiers. One of the ladies, a former schoolteacher from Leith, apparently filled a potentially awkward silence by switching the conversation to the supper menu.

Since Miranda, by then, was back at her home in Glasgow, and Victoria had homework to do, Suzi gave me a task by way of keeping troubled thoughts at bay. I was to pick up Jenni, Victoria's older sister, and the twins, who were younger, from school hockey and take them to tennis.

While I waited at the sports ground, I fielded a series of calls from my other children, Logan, Patrick and Michele, all of them wanting to know how things were going.

Jenni and the twins, when they appeared, asked a lot of questions and, young as they were, they understood. "You've done the right thing," was their reassuring message. They often referred to Norman as 'cute', which was very much the in-word of the day, however inappropriate it sounded when related to someone as belligerent as their grandfather. Yet for eighty per cent of the time at least, they had brought out the best in him. If they said he was to have a shower rather than a bath, he was far more likely to do it than if the instruction came from anyone else.

My grandmotherly tasks at an end, I headed for Tesco to buy something for my supper and some flowers to brighten up the house. It was slow going and, during a bit of a wait at the checkout, I drifted into a different world.

I came to with a start as my eye was caught by a light reflecting off the edge of the elderly checkout man's glasses. He smiled and, though I had clearly been keeping him waiting, he was polite enough to imply that he was responsible for the delay.

Back home, the first thing I saw when I opened the front door was a half-empty cup of tea on the shelf in the hall. Norman had insisted on having one more cup before we left.

I couldn't bring myself to touch it. Not then and not for another couple of days. There had been plenty of times when I had cursed under my breath at being told he wouldn't do this or that unless I made him yet another cup of tea (it used to take anything up to five cups to get him started on any article he had to write) but now I began to notice the gap. Certainly, I wasn't about to say to myself, "Thank God, I don't have to make him a cup of tea for a bit."

Next, my black cat deserted me, unfurling from her afternoon sleep and purring politely as she brushed past my legs and hurried out of the cat-flap.

It was time to put the flowers into a couple of vases, one for the lounge and the other for the porch. Half an hour later, I went back to look at the assortment in the lounge and already they were looking the worse for wear. The petals, supposedly white, looked a sorry shade of green and there was nothing cheering about them.

I watched TV for a while and, after another round of calls with all the children, I rang the home. When they said that Norman had settled down nicely, I went to bed. For the first time in years, I didn't have to worry what I did with those infernal car keys.

It had been a hard day, one of the hardest of my life, and the blatant deceit involved was probably the worst of it.

When, in the morning, the on-duty nurse told me that Norman had slept through the night without once moving from his bed, I refused to believe it. I had to check that she had the right patient. Apparently, if he had got out of bed, an alarm would have sounded, and it never did.

For my part, I had three hours' sleep in a row from ten until one followed by a nightmare. Norman was hauling a piece of heavy furniture down the stairs – it was an intricately carved Indian table – and taking it into the hall. At that moment when he started dragging it out of the house and into a neighbour's driveway, I sat up in a sweat.

I went downstairs, stroked the cat and had a drink of tea. It was hours before I got back to sleep but still that night was a vast improvement on what had gone before.

Suzi and I were going to see Norman at 2pm the following afternoon and we were each as nervous as the other.

We arrived during afternoon entertainment which involved a pretty young girl singing and playing the lute. The girl and the lute did not seem to be on the best of terms, but the girl's choice of music was good, an array of old Scottish songs. The lady from Leith, who was where she was following an operation on her knee, was sitting next to Norman and, every now and then, she tapped him on the shoulder to point something out.

Norman was not making much sense, but he had clearly established some kind of rapport with this kindly soul. He spoke to her nicely, even if his comments were in no way related to what she was saying,

As Suzi and I sat there, doing our best to contribute to this all-over-the-place conversation while not interrupting the music, Norman gave me the odd nasty stare. I wondered if he was getting his own back for what had happened the day before but, when I asked the matron if he had been asking to go back to his own home, she said he had not. She thought he did not know where he was, and that he did not mind where he was. She confirmed that he had slept through the night but added that his feet were worse than she had thought in that it had taken two people to help him get about the place. Along much the same lines, though he had initially sounded willing when someone suggested he get dressed for breakfast, he never budged and a care worker had to take charge.

Overall, the news was good and, following on from afternoon tea at the home, Suzi and I set off for Marks and Spencer where my first port of call was to buy a bunch of red and yellow tulips.

Norman was already on appropriate medication for his foot ailment, but the various tests carried out by the medical men revealed a series of more complex concerns in addition, of course, to his dementia issues. At that point, it became abundantly clear that he would not be coming home at the end of the fortnight and that he, like six other patients in much the same position, would be taking up residence in Farrow Hall.

When the time was right, Suzi, Victoria and I were asked by a staff member if we would like to go to Farrow Hall to select what we felt would be an appropriate bedroom.

My preference was for one of the few rooms with a view to the hills. Suzi and Victoria were adamant that, while it would be the right room for a lot of people, it would not be the right room for Norman. "He would sooner have a room where there was more going on outside the window," said the then 15-year-old Victoria. She was right.

The move from the first home to the second was every bit as seamless as the management predicted. Norman did not even recognise that it had happened. As far as I know, none among the six movers showed any sign of being disorientated, with the most likely explanation being that three members of staff moved with them.

Pieces of furniture were arriving at much the same time and, though the lounge could have done with a few extra tables and chairs, I learned that a grand piano was destined to fill the gap.

It was on Norman's second afternoon at Farrow Hall that he went up to the nurses' station and rang the bell as if it were hotel reception.

And that was when I had my first encounter with Alphonso, a chief nurse whose credentials included a sense of humour, something which should be a prerequisite for the lead figure in any care home. Humour apart, he had an air of authority which somehow contrived to sit well with a startling and stand-up crop of blonde hair.

"What can I do for you sir?" he asked.

"I'd like a platter," said Norman.

"Certainly, sir. Just run through what you would like it to include and I'll take a note."

Norman thought about it for a few seconds before reeling off a selection of items such as pâté and tomatoes before concluding with a bicycle.

When a smiling Alphonso returned with a cup of tea, Norman declared that it was precisely what he had wanted.

Though Norman's feet never tapped to the music when at last the piano arrived, it had nothing to do with medical matters.

Apart from enjoying a good Christmas musical such as *The Wizard of Oz* with the children and myself, he had never shown any interest in music, any more than he had ever learned to dance. Indeed, when it came to my piano-playing, he was wont to shut the door just firmly enough to make plain that the noise might interfere with whatever sport it was that he was watching on television in another room. Yet when, shortly after the Farrow Hall piano arrived, and residents and staff alike told him how much they liked the piano-playing sessions, he changed his tune.

On an afternoon when he had been delivering a series of nasty barbs, each of which had the saving grace of being as smartly delivered as you would expect of someone with his talents, he suddenly came up with a gentle query. He wanted to know how long I had been playing the piano.

"Since I was a child," I said. "Why do you ask?"

"Because I like it," he replied,

"Is there anything you like in particular?"

"I like it all."

Chapter 3: Farrow Hall

That Norman looked at ease in Farrow Hall was not surprising. This former primary school was a building he knew so well as to have taken it for granted for most of his life. In his teenage days, he passed it on his way to the local senior school and, in more recent years, it doubled as the children's primary school and a popular wine store. This historic, one-storey building was constructed from a red sandstone and boasted all of the same dependable characteristics as the other Scottish primary schools dating back to the late 1800s. These establishments had been designed to last and last they did in that you still see them everywhere, with some still serving their original purpose and others turned into offices or handsome family homes.

In its earliest years, with the stones fresh from local quarries, Farrow Hall would have looked magnificent and it was looking great again after John Marquis had owned it for a few months. Yet somewhere in its middle years, the Hall had been robbed of its charm as the local councils dumped a series of portacabins in the playgrounds. (The council must have procured a job lot because these huts were turned into tacky-looking classrooms for every primary school in the land as the population swelled.)

A more spacious local primary school was being built close to Farrow Hall and, when that was subjected to one delay after another and the original building was up for sale, the children – and they included some of my grandchildren – were ferried into Edinburgh city centre by bus. Their journey delivered them to a Dickensian place of learning which was used by a series of primary school children whose own school buildings were undergoing repairs, or being sold or extended. The bus which sallied forth to this grim alternative was always late because of the traffic, while the minute playground dictated that the pupils had to learn a new sport: hopscotch.

When John Marquis made his purchase, you would have thought that his care-home project was more of a rich man's hobby than anything else. (That opinion would be reinforced by the fact that his prices were set no higher than any of the other homes in the region.)

From the first day, everything he did to the place had to be perfect, starting with the surrounding plot of land.

The portacabins had a temporary stay of execution while serving as work stations for the men who cleaned the exterior stonework and added three accommodation wings featuring the same sandstone as the main block. And while all that was happening, an endless fleet of lorries was at the ready to make off with the latest batch of external and internal clutter before work started on the landscaping.

Architects and interior designers were consulted at every stage and Mr Marquis and his staff even called upon an expert – not a very good one or so it seemed – to suggest which fancy fish would work best in the lounge fish tank. (The fancy fish were wolfed by bigger editions.)

On to the carpets. Flecked pale blue and beige and closely woven, these were of the best quality and laid everywhere other than in the dining room, the kitchens and those areas used by visiting medical people and hairdressers. They had a soothing effect and, because they were pale, you did not have to look twice to see that they were scrupulously clean.

On those occasions when there was a spillage, it was as if the misadventure detonated an alarm. A team of maintenance men would come running and someone from somewhere would produce a piece of chalk from his or her pocket and draw a circle around the relevant patch. The same attention to detail applied to sofas and chairs.

Paintings by Constable and Lowry (people would ask in jest if they were originals) hung on the walls of the lounge, while the extravagant selection of lamps and mirrors was all in keeping with the building's age. Indeed, so understandably proud was John Marquis of his every purchase that, in passing, he was inclined to give these items the same appreciative nod as he bestowed on his paying guests.

The *pièce de résistance*, however, was the grand piano. It arrived some six months after my husband moved in and made a correspondingly grand entrance.

Though it had been polished in the showroom and the removal men had repeated the process once the instrument was in place, that was not enough for the staff at Farrow Hall. After they had overseen its arrival and shepherded it through the giant hallway and into the lounge, an eagle-eyed nurse noticed a fingerprint on the front lid and wasted no time in ringing for a duster and a tin of Pledge.

From the kitchen staff to the chiropodist, everyone came in to admire the purchase and when, finally, all their compliments had been paid, I somehow plucked up the courage to ask if I could play a tune. At first, the acting matron looked concernedly up and down the keyboard as if she were worried about further fingerprints. Only then she started to chuckle, quite possibly at herself, and decreed that it was the best of ideas.

A concert pianist I was not; I was a million miles removed from that. I gave up formal lessons while working for Grade Six but carried on playing by ear to the point where I could always reel off a miscellany of songs, old and new. For several years, and for the fun of it as much as anything else, I would play with a group of school friends at homes for the elderly in the Birmingham area.

At some point, we decided to expand our horizons and offered our services to Winson Green Prison. That the prison officer handling our enquiry asked if he could attend one of our functions before anything was agreed was seen as an exciting development. What followed, on the other hand, was anything but. His stay was brief, as was a follow-up letter in which he more or less made plain that the prisoners were deserving of something more professional.

To add to my piano-playing CV, I played in a pub in Betws-y-Coed when a friend by name of Tessa Robertson and I went hitchhiking round Wales. (It was the kind of thing sixteen-year-olds could do in the 1960s.) While I played, Tessa collected money – quite a lot of it – in a tin lent to us by the landlord.

Also worth a mention was the audition I was offered in my teens during a Christmas break spent working for that gloriously old-world store, Simpsons of Piccadilly. Staff members were asked by one of Dr Simpson's aides if anyone would like to play the piano during the shoppers' tea-time period and a couple of friends put my name forward. It was heartening when the aged manager started swaying to the music. Sadly, though, his outstretched hand at the end of my twenty-minute stint was for the purpose of delivering a consolatory ten-pound note as opposed to a congratulatory handshake which was reserved for a girl in the make-up department who was waiting to take up her place at the London Music School. (This all took place several years after Jeremy Lloyd was employed as a junior at Simpsons and drew on his experiences to pen the TV sitcom, *Are You Being Served?*)

At Farrow Hall, I played the grand piano several times a week and, after my husband's death in December 2014, I returned to the home for a few weeks while also making 'playing' visits to other care homes. The reaction to the piano seldom changed. In the case of the dementia victims, the music seemed to provide a welcome thread connecting old and present lives.

I was never on the inside to see the Coronavirus having its horrendous impact on practically every care home in the country. You can only assume that these establishments will for years to come be associated with bleak pictures of residents passing away without any relative or friend at their sides, with that image compounded by an equally disturbing vision of relatives deprived of the opportunity to bid a comforting goodbye. Yet it was during those dark times that people learned to appreciate just how much the staff in these places cared. How often did we watch TV excerpts capturing these wonderful people shedding tears at what they were witnessing? And how compelling was the following message sent to an anonymous relation of one of their Covid victims:

"*The nurses wanted you to know that your relative was not alone when they died,*" was how it began. It went on to read that they had sat with the patient and held their hand, with the words accompanied by a little box which included a wooden heart, the resident's fingerprint and a lock of hair tied with a ribbon.

More recently, there was a touching plea from one Mary Fowler, a 104-year-old Scottish care-home resident who, with the help of her daughter, took to social media to call for visiting hours during the pandemic to be eased so that she and others like her could spend more time with their relatives. Mary said that the many restrictions on visiting times had left her feeling that the home had become "like a prison". Though she thought highly of the establishment itself, she was urging people to campaign for change. "When you're my age," she said, "you deserve to see your family. Please do what you can to help. It's all you want, the happy faces around you."

To set against that sorry tale, there was one story after another of opera singers who, no longer having anywhere to sing, visited care homes to sing arias to the residents from outside the windows. What a wonderful way of adding a bit of spark to the residents' then somewhat spartan existence.

Yet long before the virus threatened the status of care homes in general, the image I had of these places was so wholly at odds with the conventional picture – one of everyone sitting, expressionless, round the room – that I had this urge to set the record straight.

As I mentioned in the introduction, I wanted people to know that the average home is not the wholly Godforsaken place that some would have us believe. Levels of sadness were often to the fore during the two and a half years during which one or more of Patrick, Suzi, Jenni, Tori, Charlotte, Jessica and I went to Farrow Hall on a daily basis and the London-based family members never failed to play their part. But the sadness, as I saw it, was seldom unremitting. In so many cases, residents' relationships with their relatives, the staff and one another was heart-warming, entertaining, uncomfortable, poignant, and sometimes all of those things. Certainly, all the care homes I visited were never short on laughter, though it was interesting to hear a friend of mine say recently that she thought people had forgotten how to laugh during the

Covid years, what with the constant stream of bad news about the pandemic, political issues and the War in Ukraine,

The reader may find there is too much of an emphasis on sport in these pages. Yet sport plays far more of a part in old age than some might think. For Norman, sport was a life-long obsession and, at Farrow Hall, he shared and spread his wealth of knowledge with his fellow residents. What information he gave them from the past would be spot on; his encouraging sign-off gambits less so. He could be talking to the oldest and frailest residents of them all but always he would advise that they would be back playing football/rugby/tennis/cricket in no time.

However improbable that was, they seemed to like the sound of it.

Chapter 4: A Wimbledon Final to Remember

It was the day of the 2013 Wimbledon final, and the residents had been ushered into the lounge. By no means all of them were entirely on the ball as to what was happening but, because this was Wimbledon and Farrow Hall seldom missed the chance to play up an occasion, the turnout was a good one. Norman, who had coached all the children at the tennis club down the garden and could play a bit himself, seemed to be looking forward to the match. Yet barely had the television been turned on that he fell asleep for the rest of the afternoon.

Nakita McBride, who scurried about the place in double-quick time and liked to give the impression that she was in charge of everyone and everything, was looking her usual self in a well-tailored grey skirt and with her hair kept firmly in place with a hairnet. Elsewhere, a couple of the ladies were clad in flowery dresses which could well have done duty in the Wimbledon stands at some point. Members of staff admired the dresses as Nakita, who said she had been named after a distant Russian relative, took it upon herself to look with contempt both on those wearing the dresses and those doing the admiring. Her mood and her manner were set for the day. Courtesy of the well-heeled gentleman who lived next door to the home, strawberries and cream were being prepared in the kitchen and, as early as half past one, glasses of elderflower cordial, apple juice and white wine were being handed round to residents and their visitors.

With Norman showing no signs of waking up, I played the theme music to the Championships before closing the piano lid and taking a seat at the back of the room. Meanwhile, Sue Barker and Tim Henman, from the ranks of the BBC commentary team, were making conversation as they waited for Novak Djokovic and Andy Murray to arrive on court.

Since their chat touched on technique, it came as no surprise when Nakita, who was peering at the television from a standing position, launched into an imaginary service action and her finishing flourish collided with

Alicia Hemple's freshly coiffured hair. Nakita looked round for approval.

"For God's sake sit down and stop making such a fool of yourself!" said Alicia, a resident who was endeavouring to regain strength in the wake of a foot operation. "I thought you were going to kill me."

While Nakita looked as if she might be considering how best to repay her sister resident for such a put-down, I asked if she had played tennis for her school. Not a good idea.

"Has no one in this place ever mentioned that I was a pretty good tennis player?" she asked. "I was the South of England champion in the 1950s and, when the family moved to Tonbridge for a while, I played in a very famous county match, the one when Kent beat Surrey. My name Nakita, incidentally, means unconquerable."

I nodded wisely before searching for a bit of support. Dorothy Smyth saved the day. Though she was late in arriving and breathless with it, she had still managed to pick up on the gist of the conversation.

"I played tennis, too," she said eagerly. "I played for St Monica's Convent in Glasgow."

Dorothy's mention of her tennis ahead of that Wimbledon final triggered a perfect example of

Nakita's brand of mischief. Instead of uttering a polite acknowledgement of her sister resident's tennis credentials, she decided at once that they needed to be put into context.

"I'm sorry, my dear, but we're not talking about school tennis. We're talking about county tennis. In any case, I don't for one minute suppose that St Monica's were any good at the sport. I know that my school in Tunbridge Wells never bothered with matches against local convents. The nuns didn't have a clue about tennis, then or now. Convent girls are probably still playing with wooden rackets for all I know."

Dorothy, a charming lady whose genteel behaviour was yet inclined to take an occasional but marked turn for the worse, was bewildered. She had told me before that she had been fond of the nuns and now she was getting tied up in knots as she tried to set the record straight. The trouble was that she was in far too much of a mental muddle to state her case.

In this instance, it did not matter overmuch. Barely had she started to fret in earnest than she was jolted by the latest camera shots on TV. The cameras were focusing on a section of the Centre Court stand where she thought that she and her husband, a one-time judge called Bernhard, used to sit on their annual Wimbledon visits. She pointed at the screen to make others aware of this development.

Nakita, to her credit, took the trouble to look. Only then she craned her head in a manner that suggested it would have been well-nigh impossible for the couple to see anything from that part of the stadium. "I'm sure your seats were fine," she said, "but my husband and I were lucky. Eric, who was high up in the army, knew someone who knew someone – the Secretary of the All England Club, as it happened – and we used to sit in the members' box. Next to the royal box, I should add."

"Oh, you were lucky," said Dorothy. "But I'm sure our tickets were satisfactory. In fact, as I remember it, we could see quite well. You don't think Bernhard would have bought cheap tickets, do you?"

"How would I know?" snapped Nakita.

Visitors exchanged uncomfortable grins. They were there to watch the final but the odd spat between Nakita and A N Other, usually added up to a diversion which could not be ignored.

A brass band had stopped playing somewhere on the grounds of the All England Club. Tim Henman and Sue Barker were winding up their pre-match deliberations and, at 14.03 precisely, Djokovic and Murray were led out on to the court.

At the same time, Alphonso, the head nurse, walked into the room with a couple of rackets under his arm. Those residents whose emotions were still in working order loved him. He made them laugh and that probably contributed rather more to their well-being than any of the pills and potions which were handed out every evening.

He turned to Nakita and Dorothy. "I hope you're backing Murray."

Nakita's face darkened at this intervention. "I don't think it's for you to tell us who we want to win. I may be more Scottish than anything else, but I prefer Djokovic. He doesn't pull as many faces. Anyhow, I lost interest in this Wimbledon when Murray beat Mikhail Youzhny. I've always kept an eye open for good Russian players. I might be related to them."

Dorothy said she was worried because she didn't know who she wanted to prevail, while her husband, who had just arrived, tried to persuade her to keep quiet.

Murray won the first set 6-4 but, in no time at all, Djokovic raced to 4-1 in the second set and Nakita was looking smug. "What did I tell you?" she said. "I knew this was how it would work out." Unfortunately for her, things promptly deteriorated from her point of view as Murray fought back to take the set 7-5, making it two sets to love.

Nakita's instincts must have dictated what she did next. While everyone else was eagerly awaiting the start of the third set, she put out her foot to bring the arriving tea trolley – it was being wheeled in by Sarah, one of the latest work-experience teenagers – to a crashing standstill. The initial thump was followed by a fountain of flying strawberries and spewing teapots.

The girl stood stock still for a few seconds before starting to pick things up, at which point Nakita advised her on the error of her ways.

"Besides making a total hash of things, you've brought this in way too soon. You need to take it back to the kitchen and bring it back in an hour or so when the match is finished." The girl seemed to be pondering on whether Nakita's orders carried more clout than the cook's and, once she had decided that they did, she wheeled the trolley out. Within a matter of seconds, she was wheeling it back.

Nakita was ready for her. "I told you to take it to the kitchen."

"The cook told me to bring it straight back in here."

"Well," returned Nakita, "you can tell the cook to go to hell."

Had the girl found herself on the set of Alice in Wonderland she could not have looked more shaken. On my bidding, she ignored Nakita and, after parking her trolley in the dining-room annex, she slumped into a chair and looked as crumpled as the oldest resident.

Barely had the match resumed than Bernhard, who had been musing out loud about the likelihood of a first British winner since Fred Perry won his third consecutive title in 1936, had to snap back into the present. Dorothy had started to snore, and Nakita let it be known, by jumping up from her seat, that every snore was affecting her well-being.

To all-round concern, Nakita left her chair altogether to go and have a word with the sleeping one. My somewhat optimistic guess was that she would do no more than alert Dorothy to the news that Murray might go on to win after all.

As it was, she gritted her teeth before giving Dorothy's shoulders a bit of a shake.

"Help, help!" cried the victim as she drooped over the right-hand side of her chair.

"Come along now, Nakita," cried Alicia Hemple. "That's not very kind." Alphonso rang an emergency button before checking that Dorothy was properly reassembled ahead of the matron's arrival.

For everyone's benefit, Nakita issued a hurried explanation.

"I shook her because she was snoring and she was ruining the tennis for the rest of us," she claimed.

Dorothy, who was now wide awake, dabbed her eyes. "I wasn't snoring," she protested.

"You were," said Nakita.

"Bring back the strawberries," called Alphonso on the recommendation of Connie, the matron. Delightfully well-organised soul that she was, Connie never overreacted to any care-home crisis. She had a quiet word with Dorothy before returning to an ailing resident in her room.

The tea trolley's second entrance was altogether less hectic. The tea and the strawberries worked their magic and everything remained quiet until Murray was leading two sets to love and 5-4 in the third set. Only by this stage, Dorothy had fallen asleep again. Cue more snores and a series of warning shots across the bows from Nakita. "Please sit down, Nakita," said Alphonso. "Hear, hear!" said Dorothy's husband and not a few others.

Nakita's anger knew no bounds at this collective telling-off. She perched herself on the edge of her seat while Murray let three match points escape and was preparing to serve for the match for a fourth time. At that key moment, she could contain herself no longer.

Seconds before Djokovic netted the backhand which would spell his defeat, she rushed up to the TV and pressed the 'off' switch. It was lucky for her that she did not find herself up against the old Norman at that stage.

In the event, it was as if rather more than the TV had come to a halt. Guests and residents alike were in a state of suspended animation to which, typically, Alphonso wasted no time in calling a halt.

"Game, set and match Nakita!" he cried.

Chapter 5: Advantage Alicia

Three days after the Wimbledon final, people were still talking about Andy Murray's win. A Dr Johnny Morton, who had watched the match at home, made his early afternoon rounds of the room-based patients before popping his head into the lounge. He wanted to hear what the residents there had to say and was sorry to learn that Norman, with his sporting credentials, was not in a position to give his views and was in any case more interested in making a return to the apple tart he had forgotten to finish at lunch.

Since Dorothy had been on the doctor's GP practice list for years (the two of them had once partnered each other in a mixed doubles match at the Bearsden Tennis Club in Glasgow) Johnny crossed the lounge to speak to her.

"What did you think of the final, Dorothy?"

"Oh Johnny," she said, "it was wonderful, absolutely wonderful. Andy got better and better as the match wore on, didn't you think?

Almost before she had finished, Nakita dived into the conversation.

"How would you know, Dorothy? You spent most of the match asleep. And you were snoring."

The doctor repressed a chuckle before making a hurried switch to Annie Lacey-Hallbright who, typically, had seen every point. Before giving her thoughts, Annie volunteered something that none of us had heard before. She had not missed a Wimbledon final – on TV or the radio – since 1953 when Maurice, the eldest of her four children, had had the decency not to be born until America's Maureen Connolly had beaten Doris Hart, another American, 8-6, 7-5. "It was a close-run thing but it worked out with five minutes to spare!"

Annie chatted to Dr. Morton about how the players seemed to hit the ball harder and harder every year. "I suppose it's something to do with the new metal rackets, though I have to say that there was never a year when I thought that they would be able to hit it harder than they already did."

Like everyone else, the doctor, who was still a regular at the local tennis club, never ceased to be intrigued by Annie's nonagenarian insights.

Alicia Hemple, another who had found the match compelling, said that she was surprised to have survived the pressure of the final. "I would have been furious if I'd passed out, or indeed on, without knowing the result." Coupled with the expression on her face, that worked as a sly crack at Nakita who had switched off the TV at that cliffhanger moment when Andy was on what turned out to be his fourth and final match point. (Alphonso had been able to put the situation to rights when, five or so minutes later, he managed to locate the replay button.)

Guy Clutterbuck, a former orthopaedic surgeon who always enjoyed talking to Jenni, the oldest of my seven grandchildren and one who had a medical career in mind, chipped in at this point. He wanted to tell the doctor that Murray would need to watch his hips if what he was hearing about his long hours of practice and training was correct. (This was 2013 and Murray went on to have hip surgery in 2019.) Dr Morton agreed. The two of them went on to discuss hip joints in general, with the doctor saying that he was seeing more and more sportsmen and women whose hips and knees were wearing out rather earlier than used to be the case. Against that, he reckoned that some people were doing more to keep fit than they had ever done.

Next to join in with the Andy Murray chat was Connie, the matron, who was returning from a long weekend. An all-round sports fanatic who went running in the hills on an almost daily basis, Matron said they should show more tennis on the TV and wondered if she should ask the management to subscribe to whatever the new channel was that was going to show all the major tennis events. "What does everyone else think about that?" she asked. Norman was the first to deliver an opinion. He thought it was possibly the best idea she had ever had.

"What are you saying?" demanded Nakita. "I think we've seen more than enough tennis in the last fortnight. In fact, if anyone mentions the name Andy Murray again, I might scream."

As it turned out, it was perfectly all right for someone else's tennis to get a mention. Namely, her own.

Later that afternoon, she took a seat about five feet away from Alicia. My piano stool made for a perfect triangle and, though my back was to the two of them, I was a happy eavesdropper.

Nakita approached her subject of choice indirectly.

"Did you play tennis, Alicia?"

"I used to play a bit but I haven't played for years," said Alicia. "I took up bowls when I was in my fifties. My husband was a keen bowler and we had this fine bowling green right across the road from us in Auchterarder. It was an obvious choice, really."

"Oh, I kept up with my tennis until I was well into my sixties," returned Nakita. "I played regular doubles in Dundee where I lived with my husband until fairly recently. One member of the four – I think her name was Lucy – couldn't play at all but I suppose it was better to have her than no one. I always used to partner Lucy because we could have a better game that way.

"Anyhow, there was one day, after she had three double-faults in a row, would you believe, that I simply had to say something. You know how it is. So I told her, 'Just serve underarm, for heaven's sake!' She took umbrage at that but it gives you an idea of just how bad she was."

"I'm surprised she wanted to go on playing with you at all after that," countered Alicia.

My grin could not be seen by either party. I had a sneaking admiration for this steely old lady who was making a slow but steady recovery from her operation. None of the other residents, bar Annie Lacey-Hallbright, was as good as she was when it came to keeping Nakita in check.

Alicia's latest riposte gave her a few minutes of welcome respite and, when Nakita started up again, she had another card to play. Out of the corner of my eye, I could see her lifting up her knitting so that it served as a shield between the two of them.

It certainly took my mind off Nakita and her tennis for a moment, for this blue and white creation-in-the-making was significantly at odds with her usual choice of colour.

Alicia tended to wear brown; a brown twin set or a brown sweater. In fact, I had this picture in my mind's eye of her bedroom drawer containing nothing but an assortment of rather dull brown knitwear and often wondered where she bought it. After all, there was seldom any sign of that shade in Marks and Spencer, or any of the other big stores for that matter.

I came to the conclusion that she must have purchased her woollens with her favourite tartan skirts in mind. She had two Campbell tartan skirts, (she had been Alicia Campbell before her marriage), with the one she had on that day a Campbell Old Weathered: a subdued but attractive mix of browns and blues.

As I signed off from one of my regular medleys, I asked her about the knitting and her face lit up to the point where it was almost as vibrant as the sweater itself. "It's for my first great grandson," she said. "His name's Jim, and everything has to be blue because the other three great grandchildren are girls."

Nakita could not be bothered with this diversion and directed the conversation back to tennis without delay.

"Funnily enough, my Kent county team used to play in blue and white sweaters in those days. And the blue was the same shade that you're using now."

"Really!" said Alicia, who had made the mistake of putting the knitting back on her lap for a moment.

"Yes, really. I expect I've still got it somewhere, because I distinctly remember wearing it when I played in an Over-45s match in Monaco where we played against the local team following an invitation from Prince Rainier. We were using the same courts where they play the Monte Carlo Masters and I certainly didn't disgrace myself. I played at No. 1 for our side –

my name, Nakita, means 'unconquerable', as I've probably told you – and I beat their best player, a Melanie du Pontier, 6-3, 6-3. She took it well considering she hadn't lost a match that season up until then.

"After the tennis we attended a grand ball. Everything's so grand out there, you know. I even got to dance with the Prince. A waltz I remember."

That triggered another less-than-convincing "Really!"

"Have you ever met royalty, Alicia?"

"Actually, I have."

"Who, exactly?"

"The Duchess of Kent."

"Oh, she's one of the few members of our royal family I haven't met. I've tended to meet the more senior royals. The Queen Mother came to our Village Institute fair once on her way down from Balmoral and she bought two jars of my blackberry jam. I also met the Queen when my husband received his MBE at the Palace. That was a lovely day!"

I delayed embarking on a fresh round of tunes for long enough to see Alicia looking heavenwards while managing to say that it must indeed have been a lovely day.

It was enough to encourage Nakita to keep the conversation alive.

"So you didn't say where you met the Duchess?"

"At Wimbledon, actually."

"At Wimbledon?"

"Yes, Wimbledon."

"Did she suddenly appear on that main walkway in front of the scoreboard or something? I know that she and the Duke of Kent used to come out and talk to very ordinary members of the public from time to time. In fact, I've even seeing her stopping to talk to people in the ticket queue."

"No," said Alicia. "I didn't see her on the walkway and I didn't see her in the ticket queue. She came on to the centre court to give me a medal."

"You, a medal? What on earth for?"

"I'd played in an exhibition mixed doubles for the Armed Forces."

While I was in silent awe at what Alicia was saying, Nakita's mind was working overtime, though not for long.

"Personally," she said, "I could never be bothered with mixed doubles."

Chapter 6: A Lesson

A student called John, who was on his way to becoming an optometrist, was spending a week in Farrow Hall as one of his work experience assignments. Since he was only going to be at the home for five days, no one had given him chapter and verse concerning the different patients; his brief was too simple for that. All that was expected of him was to spend quality time with the people on the ground floor and to get a rough picture of what was involved.

On his first day, this easy-going Irishman did what Norman told him to do in apprising him of what sports he had played and where. Once he had complied with that line in questioning by saying that he had been "a so-so footballer", John joined a couple of ladies who were sitting between Norman and the piano and, when they made clear that theirs was a private conversation, he moved on to Maggie McDougall. The latter was an eighty-something-year-old with dire arthritis, who was sitting on the piano's far side.

As a rule, Maggie kept herself to herself. She was not a regular member of the inner set who sat in the 'dress circle' seats in front of the TV. Instead, she spent most of her days in the corner, comfortably ensconced behind her copy of *The Scotsman*. The various goings-on in the room were neither here nor there as far as she was concerned.

In my first week of playing the piano on a more regular basis, when I asked if there was any tune she would like to hear, she told me that if her mother was in the room, she would want "something Scottish". So that is what I gave her. She thanked me nicely at the end of it, though I got the impression that one tune was enough.

Maggie had an occasional companion in the lounge in the person of Professor Margaret Mary Perkins, a centenarian jigsaw addict, and another newspaper reader. Though the two of them shared this kindred interest, they rarely spoke beyond reading out the front-page headlines in their respective journals. It was a quaint if delightful little ritual which both saw as a more-than-adequate level of socialising.

However, the arrival of John showed Maggie in a new light. She fell into easy chat with this good-looking young Irishman and, once he mentioned what he was doing at Farrow Hall and how he was training to be an optometrist, there was no stopping the two of them. "I wanted to be one of those," she told him. She quizzed him about the various aspects of his course, with the first of the many questions pertaining to when he first started to peer into people's eyes as opposed to picking everything up from a textbook.

"Good question," said John, before introducing a light-hearted twist to his answer. "I've always looked into my girlfriend's eyes a lot but, when it comes to what's on the university curriculum, there's not too much in the way of 'live' peering in the first couple of years. I'm sure it's different at other universities, but I'm at Plymouth where it's not until your third year that you work with real eyes and real patients. The university has its own eye-care centre of excellence, which helps."

Maggie told John he had made a wise choice of career. Her questions ceased for a couple of minutes as she regaled him with details of how she had made regular visits to the opticians as a small child because she, like her mother, was short-sighted. "I had glasses, but I didn't really wear them when I was young because I didn't want to be the only child in my class wearing spectacles. So I probably made my eyes worse. What's more, I've got a daughter, Karen, who ended up making the same mistakes I did. Anyhow, I've spent a lot of time over the years wondering about the best way to get children to wear glasses. What do you think?"

John said he was still learning, but he thought an optician could play a large part in making a young patient see his or her glasses in a positive light. "It's different for boys, I think. Most of them seem to like the look of themselves in spectacles."

Maggie was relentless with her queries and John, in turn, was enjoying finding someone who was genuinely fascinated in what he was doing. Eventually, though, she began to tire and, as that happened, so she went off-piste. Like many of the Farrow Hall patients, male and female, she started mentioning her mother. "She's upstairs, you know. Do you think I should go and find her? I'd like to see how she's getting on."

From what I could hear, John was dealing with the situation with admirable tact. "I'm sure she's fine," he said, "but the people upstairs are getting their supper earlier than we do down here at the moment, so I don't know that now's a good time. The staff will be run off their feet." (He was obviously from the Alphonso school of thought in saying something which was not likely to make her fret.)

"You're probably right," said Maggie. "I should have thought to ask sooner."

She nodded off at that point and John spoke with a few more of the residents before signing off for the evening.

Maggie McDougall's face lit up the next day when John came her way again. Without anything in the way of an opening gambit about the weather or the unusually tasty apple tart which had been on the lunch menu, she ploughed straight into more important matters. "What's the biggest changes you're seeing in eye treatment?"

"Good heavens," said John. "Let me think about that for a second; it's a tough question you're asking." He closed his eyes for a bit before coming up with what sounded like an acceptable answer. "Well," he began, "the equipment is getting more advanced all the time and it's tough to keep up to speed. In the old days, as you'll know, the patients seemed to do little more than look at one of those charts where the letters get smaller and smaller. Now, there are machines which click, flash and ping and do all the hard work. Every day it seems that there's some fascinating new development. You'd be amazed."

The above conversation was taking place at the same time as Norman was starting on a post-lunch snooze. I sat down with the two of them for a bit and noted how the moment Maggie started to tire, the same thing happened as on the previous day: she started talking about her mother. The refrain was much the same: "I know she's upstairs, but what do you think she's doing now?"

Annie Lacey-Hallbright, whose arrival had turned us into a party of four, helped John out. "I think she'll be having a good old chin-wag with my mother," she said, which, by my reckoning, would have made her mother somewhere between 110 and 120. Maggie gave Annie a kindly pat on the hand as she replied, "You're probably right, Annie." Problem solved.

The third and fourth days of John's secondment were no different and just as arresting. Lots more interesting 'eye' chat, this time about a cataract operation Maggie had had ten or so years before. That topic was spread across two afternoons and, on each occasion, ended up where John had anticipated, with references to her mother. On the Thursday John steered the chat to his own mother long enough to have her nodding off and, on the Friday, he said that the upstairs contingent – there were 17 of them altogether – were watching a film. "I'd take you up there now, but they've dimmed the lights, so I don't think we'd be able to see who's watching and who isn't."

"Well, if that's the case, it's probably better if we leave them to it," said Maggie. She was yawning at that point, but the mention of films had her stirring. "I can't think, incidentally, why we don't get more films down here."

"You get live piano," said John. "I think you're lucky."

To my relief, for I had never been able to gauge whether Maggie liked the piano sessions or not, her reply was positive. "Actually," she said, "I prefer the piano any day. The only thing is that it makes me wish I'd been better at reading music."

"Maybe you should have kept wearing those glasses!" said John.

"My mother would agree with you," she said.

That day, she expanded on the topic of her somewhat dominant mother and how she used to take a school ruler to her fingers if she failed to concentrate on her piano scales. Another thing which loomed large in the daughter's memory was how the mother used to make her stand on a dining-room table for hours on end while she straightened the hem of her school skirt. Maggie had to turn round and round to the point where she felt dizzy, sick and shattered. That, in turn, reminded her of school picnics in the Malvern Hills. On such occasions, her mother would dispatch her with enough kit for a weekend away. Though the picnic she prepared was always a good one, it would be ruined by the amount of accompanying baggage, which included gumboots, waterproofs, a woolly hat and a complete change of clothing. Since the coach driver insisted that nothing should be left in the coach, all bags had to be lugged round by their owners for the entire afternoon.

That, though, was more or less it for days three and four.

Had I been assessing John's performance for his tutors, I would have given him full marks. His sheer charm made him a winner with all the residents. Indeed, he had even passed the ultimate test by having a smiling conversation with Professor Perkins.

On his fifth and final day, John went to each of his new friends to say his goodbyes. He went from Annie to Nakita, to Dorothy, and then to Maggie. Only while he and Maggie were in mid-conversation – about eyes, of course – there was a rude interruption as a bundle of fury arrived by wheelchair. Mandy, the care-home assistant, was at the controls as she fielded a series of impatient instructions from the passenger. "Over there, not here! For heaven's sake, can't you listen? Haven't you ever pushed a wheelchair before? I want to be in front of the television and facing the room."

No one in the room complained. They just waited, politely, to see what on earth this visitation was all about.

Like an ancient weighing machine taking a few seconds to arrive at its verdict, the wheelchair lady flapped her hands round and round before finishing up with a long, lean finger pointing directly at Maggie.

"So there's Maggie," she announced to the room at large. "Would you believe that she's been too busy all week to come upstairs and see her old mother."

Maggie cringed. Only John cringed more.

He turned to me as Maggie struggled to her feet to give her mother a kiss. "Why, oh why, didn't anyone tell me?"

"I'm so sorry," I said, "but I didn't know."

Chapter 7: A Mixed Club

New male residents were a bit of a rarity and this was the first morning that the latest arrival had appeared in the lounge. He wore a freshly-pressed navy blazer, a spanking white shirt, a club tie – I couldn't tell which club – and one half of a pair of old leather brogues. His left foot was in a black boot, presumably because of a break of some sort.

Colonel Johnson-Edwards, whose hair was a greying version of Boris Johnson's untamed locks only a tad tidier, looked round the room before fixing his stare on the two women, Alicia and Nakita, who happened to be sitting in front of the television and enjoying a cup of tea. I guessed that he was irritated that they should be occupying the best seats in the house when a replay of some famous Manchester United match was about to start.

After a couple of noisy tuts which doubled as the sign-off notes from my latest batch of tunes, he asked

Norman if he knew why the women were there and when Norman described them as 'members', he stormed out of the door, walking stick outstretched as opposed to serving its supposed purpose. He was looking for Alphonso and, fortunately for the new arrival, for he looked as if he might keel over at any moment, the ever-cheerful Alphonso appeared like a genie and took his arm.

"What can I do for you, Colonel?"

"If you come into the room, you'll see for yourself," said the Colonel.

"Aha! I think you want to sit in front of the TV."

"You're wrong. I'm not interested in the football, or at least this game. I follow Liverpool. It's the women that are worrying me. There's two of them."

"Only two?"

The Colonel was irritated at what he took to be an unnecessarily facetious comment from a member of staff.

"What I want to know is why, when it's the men's lounge, are there any women in here at all? I was told that this place was run along the same lines as my golf club up the road and it looks suspiciously to me as if that's not the case."

"Well," said Alphonso, "we've always taken women. In fact, I think that most of the golf clubs in the area nowadays take them, too, don't they?"

"Well, they certainly don't at my place along the coast. I have every intention of voting against letting them in if and when the time comes."

"And why is that?

The Colonel was verging towards the apoplectic.

"I get the impression that you don't play golf, young man."

"Actually," said Alphonso, "I do. Very badly, I grant you, but I can certainly play a bit."

"Probably not enough. If you even had half a clue as to what the game was about, you'd know that women are a darned nuisance on the course. They're painfully slow because they never stop chatting and they can't hit the ball out of their shadows. The other thing I have against them is that they are hopeless at finding their golf balls when they dribble them into the rough. I think they expect other people to look for them half the time."

He took a necessary breather at that point and perched himself on the wing of an otherwise empty chair.

"I wouldn't sit there if I were you," said Alphonso. "It's safe enough but it worries me. Let me help you switch to this sofa over here so that I can hear the rest of your story."

"It's annoying that you interrupted me," said the Colonel, as he sank into the cushions. "I've lost track of what I was saying."

"You were complaining about the women. Something to do with them losing golf balls in the rough."

"Yes, that's right. Well, what I was going to add was that I think it's a darned good idea that they're thinking of altering the game's rules to say that you can only search for a ball for three minutes rather than five. I don't know when that's going to happen [it happened in 2019] but it can't happen soon enough as far as I'm concerned."

Alphonso called me across. I was in mid-tune while finding the golf conversation rather more interesting than whatever it was I was playing.

"You're a golfer, aren't you, Mrs Mair? What do you think of what the Colonel is saying?"

It was a pity Norman wasn't awake for he would have had his tuppence-worth. As it was, he was tired following a visit from the grandchildren, Olivia, Venetia and Alex, who had come up from England with their mother, Rachel.

Since I had no desire to get involved in the conversation, I suggested to Alphonso that he would do better to defer to a lady called May Simpson who, like him, had taken up short-term residence in Farrow Hall after a rather nasty fall. That very day, I had learned that May had won three Scottish championships in her golfing heyday.

The Colonel looked alarmed.

"Did I hear you say the name May Simpson?"

"You did."

"Well," he conceded, "I have to admit that May Simpson could play a bit. Oddly enough, she won the Scottish Women's championship at Fillin Hill in the year that I was involved with the Scottish Golf Association and was given the job of handing over the trophy. She's not still playing, is she?"

I did not know the answer to that one.

"Not at the moment she isn't," chipped in Alphonso. "She's like you. She's had a bad fall and she's staying with us until she's a bit steadier on her feet."

"Staying here?"

"Yes. If you look behind those chairs, she's the one sitting in front of the doors leading into the garden. She's got one foot up on a stool."

Alphonso glanced at his watch. It was three o'clock. "May likes to be woken around now so I'll take you to meet her."

"No thanks. Maybe later."

"Sorry, I can't do later. I'm off duty in twenty minutes. We'll just go now if that's all right."

Alphonso helped the Colonel to stand up, which was a difficult task when the gentleman didn't want to budge and, a couple of minutes later, the two of them were at May's side.

"Excuse me, May. I have someone here who knows you from your golfing days. He says he presented you with one of your trophies."

So flustered did the Colonel look at this point that I could only imagine that he was hoping against hope that May Simpson could not remember the first thing about the occasion. Unluckily for him, she boasted one of the finest memories in the house. And, still more unluckily, she was decidedly deaf and spoke very loudly.

She opened her eyes and looked up. Her stare was long and hard and her voice an anger-fuelled boom.

"I know him all right, Alphonso. I don't suppose he told you that he lost to me in a women's versus men's match at Hillspindle after he had to present me with that trophy. He was far and away the rudest golfer I'd ever met. Didn't even congratulate me when I holed out of a bunker at the 15th. In fact, I thought I heard him call me 'a lucky cow' though I don't suppose he's ever admitted to it. In this day and age, it would amount to abuse and maybe even now it's not too late to sue him! She paused as one who was mulling over the idea before returning to her story.

"We were both at the top table at a big dinner that night, and, all the way from the hors d'oeuvre to an excellent treacle pudding, he never spoke a word – at least to me he didn't.

"So now, if you don't mind, I'm going to go back to sleep."

"Well, that's telling you!" said Alphonso, as he steered the terrified Colonel back to his room.

Colonel Johnson-Edwards had been in hiding for a good half an hour when his daughter, Marjorie Anderson, arrived for her first visit.

Having scanned the lounge to no avail, she came across to introduce herself when I was examining my up-to-date list of tunes. (On a journey up to the Highlands to interview a golf club secretary, I had added a couple more after listening to a medley of Frank Sinatra numbers. 'As Time Goes By', was one, 'Blue Moon' another.)

Marjorie, for that is what she asked to be called, was a delight. She talked about how much she liked the look of the home as somewhere her father would be safe for the next few months while she was working at a research centre in China. Again, a key factor in the family's choice of establishment had been the astroturf putting green which had been laid down beyond the car park. Marjorie was sure that it would be well-used by her curmudgeonly old father. "You see," she said, "I told him that this place would be rather like his golf club and that there would be people here with whom he would have plenty in common."

I failed to restrain a chuckle.

"I'm afraid that your father has decided that it's not at all like his golf club. He's discovered that we take women."

"Oh dear! Did he notice?"

"I'm afraid he did. He couldn't believe that there were a couple of them in here this morning – apart from myself, that is – and then I did the wrong thing by asking him if he knew of a woman golfer called May."

The colour drained from Marjorie's face. "Not May Simpson for heaven's sake? Please don't tell me she's staying here. He was so disgracefully rude to the poor woman when she beat him some years ago that I don't think anyone's ever forgotten. Personally, I think he should have been stripped of his position with the Scottish Golf Association."

"Well," I said, "she certainly got her own back earlier this afternoon. When Alphonso thought that he and May might like to renew their acquaintance, May told him exactly what she thought of him."

Marjorie stood there, smiling and cringing at the same time. "You know what, my dad mentions her name so often that I've always wondered if he would welcome a chance to apologise."

"Well let's give him that chance," I said. "Why don't you go and fetch him from his room and the three of us can join her for tea."

Marjorie, a no-nonsense type, disappeared and returned a few minutes later dragging her grim-faced father behind her. Apparently, she had told him that the first thing he needed to do was to shake May Simpson by the hand and say he was sorry for his behaviour all those years ago.

In the event, to Marjorie's surprise and mine, he did all of that before adding a rather disarming little joke. "I've grown up a bit since then," he told her. "I'm ninety-two, now."

The ice was broken and, before too long, Marjorie and I were superfluous to requirements.

After the pair had compared notes on their recent falls – May had tripped over one of those vintage little leather golf bags in her hall cupboard and the Colonel had been knocked over by a neighbour's over-friendly Alsatian – the conversation turned to golf. The old man wanted to know what club May had used for her approach at the second hole in their match of fifty or so years before. A six-iron, apparently; she remembered it well because she had taken aim on a particular slope on the green and the ball had rolled unerringly towards the hole.

"The putt I had left was only fifteen inches or so, but you were rude enough to ask me to hole it," she remembered.

"I'm so sorry," he muttered before hurriedly plying her with a request which was less likely to make trouble.

"I'd love to know how you used to hold your putter."

At that, she rose from her chair and turned one of her walking-sticks the wrong way up. "This will do," she said, eyeing it as critically as she might a spanking new club.

She lined up the hooked handle on the carpet before replicating her old putting stroke as best she could, bearing in mind her unsteady stance.

The Colonel looked on admiringly. As soon as May was back in her seat, he took the risk of quizzing her about the bunker shot he had deemed so lucky. She desisted from repeating what he had called her at the time and began on a description of how the ball had been half-buried in the sand. The Colonel, it seemed, could not wait to hear more, only then the chiropodist arrived to say that May was the next on his list, which was why she had had no option but to bring their conversation to a halt.

She stood up and assembled her walking sticks before promising the Colonel that she would resume her account of how she had played the shot over dinner.

Only after she had made her way to the all-purpose little surgery across the corridor did the Colonel turn his attention back to Marjorie and myself.

"You know what," he said. "I think May knows more about the golf than any of my old cronies at the club."

Chapter 8: Moments

Annie Lacey-Hallbright, a sprightly nonagenarian if ever there were one, was her usual busy self. When one of her fellow residents called for help to get up and go to the bathroom, this friendly lady would scurry out of the lounge to inform a member of staff. The staff were inclined to view her as an extra pair of hands and, though visiting inspectors might well have been tempted to mark the home down because of Health and Safety concerns, or something along those lines, Annie revelled in her role.

On 13 May 2013, Annie had performed more than her usual quota of good deeds and decided to give herself a break. She drew a chair up next to the piano stool and asked for a couple of tunes before I signed off to join Norman for the morning coffee break. Her tunes of choice were as old as she was herself – 'I Love Paris, Lily of Laguna' and 'She'll Be Coming Round the

Mountain' – and, when I had signed off from that little selection, she stayed on for a chat.

In her youth, Annie had been a French teacher on the Isle of Lewis before moving to the mainland after her marriage to a Church of Scotland minister. You could see from the twinkle in her eye that teaching was a job she had loved and, all these years later, she could still have helped young children with their early French. In fact, I once heard her helping a work-experience schoolgirl with her Higher French grammar.

She was sharp beyond belief and, to give just one illustration, everyone who came to the home, be they visiting medical people, visitors, or other residents, would look with admiration on how she was usually to be found dashing through a book of advanced crosswords. Little by little, though, she had been forced to accept that it was probably for the best that she had moved to Farrow Hall from her pretty cottage in a row of what used to be mill workers' cottages down by the river. Her children had become concerned lest she repeat a series of adventures in which she had taken off on one of her endless walks and ended up in a different neighbourhood. A consignment of family members and friends had been sent out on each occasion and she had felt guilty for making a nuisance of herself.

The only time I ever saw Annie out of sorts was in connection with her love of walking.

It was on a fresh, early spring morning that she looked into the lounge – she was dressed in a camel coat and a fetching pink beret – and announced she was going out.

"Where are you off to, Annie?" asked Marie Mason, a kindly nurse from the Highlands.

"I'm off for a walk, only I'm having a bit of bother with the front door," said the old lady. "It appears to be locked. *Je suis tres ennuyé!*"

Marie, who did not need to have studied French to understand Annie's finishing gambit, stuttered a bit over her reply. "Let's, er, go and give the door a try but, if there's a problem, why don't we wait till someone can go with you. It's not that nice outside you know."

Annie's brow began to furrow. "I don't want to wait for anyone to come with me, thank you very much. I want to go walking on my own, just as I've done for the last fifty years and, to be honest, I don't care about the weather. And by the way, since I'm paying to be here, I think I should be allowed to do as I like. I'm not a prisoner, after all."

The nurse had buzzed for Connie, the matron, and now the latter arrived and set about trying to make the resident believe that she could have her own way. Of course she could go for a walk, but would she mind showing the new nursing assistant the whereabouts of the post office?

As Annie looked her in the eye, you could see that she was not impressed. "There may be people in this home who might fall for that but I'm not one of them I'm afraid," she said. She then took a long enough break to be sure that her reproach had sunk in before adding a more gently styled addendum. If, on the off-chance that what the matron was saying was not a ruse, she would take the girl with her.

Annie and the nursing assistant became as old friends that morning, probably because the occasion made for an inviting little escape for both. They were away for a good three-quarters of an hour and, on their return, they reported that they had met some unexpected newcomers in the field below the woods: some magnificent highland cows. To Annie's delight, their owner brought one of them across to make her acquaintance and she had asked, in jest, if she could cut its fringe.

Even if she was back to her old happy and inspiring self by the end of that outing, the events of the morning had shown very clearly that this much-loved resident had been sorely shaken at the realisation that she could no longer go where she wanted, when she wanted.

For a similarly rude awakening, there was an Italian gentleman, Costantino Dassu, who adhered to the pattern of daily life with a studied calm until a day came when he set off down the corridor with an unusually purposeful stride. Every now and then, he would stop to give a drummer-like swirl of a handsome walking-stick which, he had told me, was carved from fine Indian rosewood. His brother had bought it for their elderly father when he was out in the Punjab looking for herbs and spices to import for the grocery store he had planned to open on Princes Street.

Finally, he came to a full stop in front of the first of a series of seven pictures of Old Edinburgh and the Borders which were the home-owner's pride and joy. He had selected them himself and they included one from the opening day of the Forth Road Bridge in the Fifties, and another featuring the last day of the original trams which had been part of the Edinburgh landscape from 1871 to 1956.

On the day that Costantino Dassu had his moment of revelation, he was in no mood for happy reminiscences. Instead, in what was a rather more extreme version of Annie's flash of anger, he looked long and hard at the first of those pictures – some serenely grazing horses in a Border field – before smashing the glass with his walking-stick. He then moved on to apply the same treatment to the second and third pictures, by which time the home's maintenance team were in hot pursuit.

"What's the matter, Costantino?" said Sarah, the teenage work-experience girl who had been at the centre of the Wimbledon tea-trolley debacle.

"I want to go home," he said.

Sarah risked being the next victim of the walking-stick treatment as she put a friendly arm round the resident. "But this is your home."

"We both know that it isn't," said Costantino.

Having got that much off his chest, he sat down and enjoyed a cup of coffee, all as if nothing had happened.

During the course of my coffee-time chat with Annie, I mentioned that I had seen a notice announcing that the local bowling club was looking for people of all ages who would be interested in giving the sport a try or simply watching one of their matches. I asked if she would like me to take her to see what went on behind the club's high hedges and, for a moment, I thought she was going to answer in the affirmative.

"I'm tempted," she said, "and it's very kind of you to ask. I used to play bowls or '*Pétanque*', as everyone called it when we went to Provence on family holidays. But the thing is that you don't really want to be bothered with anything like that in your nineties."

She glanced up, seemingly in the expectation that I would carry the conversation forward. I waited until I was sure of that before asking, "So what do you want from life at this stage?"

Predictably, she did not answer until she had given the matter a bit of thought.

"Well, as you know," she began, "I like a good walk but, beyond that, I really don't want very much. I'm happy here and I'm happy that my sons and daughters don't have to worry about me. If I weren't happy, they would be worried and that would be upsetting.

"There are odds and ends you have to sort out for yourself, but I don't look for things to do. If things are happening here, I join in. I come to all the fitness classes and I'll come along when there's a good movie on the television, when there's a craft class, or when I hear the piano. I've always been like that. I can't be bothered with people who are always complaining about being old. It's been happening since the beginning of time and I often wonder why we've not got used to the idea of getting on with what's left of our lives and making the most of those years. It's by no means all bad!"

After a bit more thought, she volunteered that she liked the food at Farrow Hall. "You never know what's coming but it's all good. I've never heard anyone complain. In fact, I'm thinking now that there's a slight whiff of the Ratatouille which I noticed was on the supper menu. I'm just hoping I put my tick beside that rather than the omelette. It's not that I dislike omelettes, it's just that they can be a little boring."

While Annie reminded the approaching chiropodist that her appointment was not until the following week, I glanced across at a woman at the far end of the room, Agatha James, whose manner was the antithesis of Annie's. As far as I could tell, she specialised in being gloomy and polished the art every time her daughter, Corinne, came to visit.

Corinne, a part-time executive at an Edinburgh hotel, let her enjoy the process. Every day, she would make a two-mile round trip to listen to her mother's litany of woes, with the main positive – apart from the fact that she was salving her conscience – that she was able to make good progress on the hat she was knitting. For her mum.

She chuckled at the more acerbic of her mother's asides and, much to my amazement, the same applied even after she had broached the subject of how she and her husband would be going to Lisbon one weekend.

At that, the mother raised her head to deliver the ultimate in monstrous declarations: "I'll be dead by the time you get back."

Corinne's reaction was to pass it off as if her mother had said nothing more significant than that her cup of tea might be cold by the end of the trip. She did, though, go on to mention how their cousin, John, would be coming in to see her on the Sunday.

"How could you do that to me?" demanded Agatha. "You know I can't stand John."

"Not to worry. I'll tell him to bring you some strawberries."

"Tell him not to bother."

At that, Annie, standing nearby, was moved to intervene.

"Tell him to give them to me," she said.

Corrine laughed and, though I am probably getting a bit carried away, I would like to think that the mother had to struggle not to do the same.

Annie, when I last saw her in the winter of 2019, was 101 and still going strong. One of her sons, Pierre, was taking her to a quaint little coffee shop near the seafront at Portobello – a well-nigh impossible task in that there was nowhere to park on the coffee shop's side of the road.

I ran into the two of them as they were walking arm in arm along the pavement opposite and they paused for a chat.

The three-way conversation was still in full flow when Annie, who had been burrowing in her handbag for her watch, gave it a swift check before apologising profusely. She said that she would need to drag Pierre away because it was 10 o'clock and she had a hair appointment at midday back at Farrow Hall.

They crossed the road and, as Pierre opened the door of the café to let Annie in first, he turned to give me a wink. It was a wink to cover what we were both thinking. Namely, that his mother's ongoing competence knew no bounds.

Chapter 9: Save the Last Dance for me

The story of Betsy Aspley-Devine and her husband Henry was well known at Farrow Hall. The couple had danced their way round the world in their sixties and seventies, mostly on cruise ships, but also at a selection of top hotels where dancing to some famous band was a feature of the evening entertainment. When prizes were handed out, this handsome couple had usually been in the running. Their foxtrot, according to visiting relatives, had been out on its own and, back in the early 1990s, they won a weekend at London's Grosvenor House Hotel where they danced to the strains of the Glen Miller Orchestra.

During one of his daily visits to see Betsy at Farrow Hall, Henry told me how they had met on the dance floor when they were in their early twenties. He had been a member of the Young Farmers' Association in Hawick but, to Norman's irritation, had not doubled that with a membership of the town's rugby club. As for Betsy, she was the daughter of one of the town's doctors. The couple did not know each other from school because Betsy had gone to an all-girls' establishment, but both had been dispatched by their mothers to Susan Rutherford's School of Ballroom Dancing at one time or another. Henry said that during their very first dance, he had recognised Rutherford touches in Betsy's footwork and she in his. They had fallen into step in every sense, and nothing had changed thereafter, not just on the dance floor but in life itself.

For thirty years after their marriage in 1958, they divided their time between farm work and bringing up their four children – two sons and two daughters. But when it came to the 1990s and their sons, John and Peter, were sufficiently experienced to run the farm on their own, the couple went along with a suggestion that they join a couple of their oldest friends on a Mediterranean cruise which focused on fine dining and dance.

Henry laughed at the memory of his sons' blank stares when he told them they would be gone for three weeks. And when John, the older of the two, asked, "Who's going to do the early morning milking?" he had his answer at the ready: "You'll need to decide that between the two of you."

You could tell from Henry's bemused smile that he held nothing against either of them. "To be honest," he told me, "they're good lads and always have been. It's just that they didn't seem to understand what Betsy and I had been doing all those years. Mind you, they learned pretty quickly! Once we had taken off on that cruise, we went on one dancing holiday after another, sometimes to our favourite hotel in Singapore and sometimes to Hong Kong. We even danced our way to New York and back on the Queen Mary in the late 1990s." Mostly, they went with those same old friends but, if they were not available, the Aspley-Devines were happy to go on their own and make new ones.

Henry's recollections of those dancing days were twenty years in the past when, while Betsy dozed in her chair, he sat back at Farrow Hall and told me of the changes in his wife which had first started to become apparent in 2009. She had taken to going downstairs in the small hours of the morning, turning on taps and gas fires and forgetting to turn them off again. That much he had been able to keep to himself but when, a year or so on, she released a party of pigs in the small hours of the morning, he had to accept that things were getting out of hand. The pigs had given the game away by behaving in rumbustious fashion in a neighbour's garden.

All four of the Aspley-Devine children had received first-hand accounts from the neighbour in question and when, a couple of weeks later, Betsy disappeared altogether (she had joined a party of students on a late-night bus to Glasgow) the children put a collective foot down.

They told Henry that his "dilly-dallying", as they called it, had to stop. Betsy was at a stage where she would need to go into a home for his sake as much as hers and, though Henry protested vehemently at the outset, he soon admitted that he was struggling to cope.

Henry paused at this moment to check that Betsy was still snoozing. She was and, since she continued to look at peace with the world, so her doting husband felt able to resume. "Since Betsy's cousin had been in one of the Farrow Hall's sister homes for a bit, I drove her down to look at that place and then this. She preferred this one from the moment she saw it and, when I asked if she would like to stay here while I flew over to France to see an ailing sister of mine, she jumped at the chance. She was under the impression that it was a cruise ship and said she would need to buy a couple of new dresses for the stay. Since she moved in, she's never wanted to leave."

No one took greater pains than Betsy with regard to dressing in the mornings. Henry had packed one of those massive old army-green trunks with a selection of her favourite clothes and, first thing every morning, she would sort out an outfit appropriate to what was on Farrow Hall's latest schedule. On Tuesdays, when I was usually at the piano, she would don one of her finest dresses, with her favourite taffeta affair in blue-green which she teamed with pretty blue shoes.

She was wearing it one Tuesday in November 2013 when the atmosphere at Farrow Hall was as good as it gets. Merry chatter was competing with the music and all the residents and their visitors were nicely relaxed. Only when I played 'You Make Me Feel So Young' and people were in full foot-tapping mode, Henry began to show signs of restlessness. This strong man rose from his seat and set about shoving hefty chairs – and not a few startled residents – to the edge of the wooden square in the centre of the room.

The moment I sensed what was on his mind, I started on the introduction to that Frank Sinatra number again. At that, he gave me a wink before making his way over to fetch Betsy. He reached for her hand and she knew at once what awaited.

As they set off across the floor, I had no trouble in picturing what an arresting couple they must have made in their finest dancing years. Though Henry looked every inch a rugged, weather-worn farmer, the years melted away with the music and he was all elegance. Betsy, a comfortably-contoured woman, was blessed with rather more than an easy style and nifty footwork. She had the kindest of smiles and, only the previous day, I had heard the yoga teacher say that she would love to look as good as she did when she was in her eighties.

For well-nigh ten minutes, the couple danced their way back into their glorious past, with Henry inordinately proud as he twirled and swirled his wife around the floor in front of a fast-growing audience. One professional move blended seamlessly with another and the performance, which ended with a kiss, said everything about the affection they had for each other.

Residents, visitors and nurses alike were visibly moved and, as Henry delivered his radiant spouse back to her seat, everyone broke into a round of applause which I can hear to this day. One or two members of staff could only dab at their eyes.

Henry was looking tired and somewhat melancholy when it was time for him to go back to his lonely farmhouse but, before he left, he came across to thank me. "That was such a happy little interlude for Betsy and myself. It took us back to the good old times so I can't thank you enough."

I said that I should be thanking him. "You made my day, Henry. In fact, I think you made everyone's day."

He asked if he could put in a request for the following Tuesday, the next of my piano-playing afternoons and Betty's eighty-first birthday. Was there any chance that I would be able to play her favourite song, 'Dancing Cheek to Cheek' from *Top Hat*, famously danced by Fred Astaire and Ginger Rogers in the Thirties.

"Pretty much," I said. "but I can make sure I know it well by next week."

I played it over and over during the next few days and tried it out on the twins, Charlotte and Jessica, before telling them the story of Henry and Betsy. They asked if they could come along to hear the birthday rendition.

When the day arrived, the three of us waited with bated breath for the couple to appear. Would they want to dance again? What would Betsy be wearing?

With no sign of them after the first half hour, I went to Matron's office to check that all was well.

"Is Betsy all right?" I asked.

The matron's expression was grave.

"Betsy's fine but I'm sorry to have to tell you that I've just had a call to say that Henry's dead."

"Henry's dead?" I repeated. "Whatever happened?"

"He rang one of his daughters early yesterday evening and told her he was tired and that he was planning on an early night as he wanted to be at his best on the dance floor for today. So he went to bed early and he never woke up."

"But he always looked so healthy. Was there anything specifically wrong with him?"

"Take your pick. The doctors said it was a heart attack; I say it was a broken heart."

Chapter 10: Lost and Found

Losing things can be catching and one late July morning Norman was the first to set the trend in motion. It may have been down to the Wimbledon fortnight, or more likely the scent of freshly-mown grass outside the open window which had him thinking of the whereabouts of his old Dunlop racket.

James, a teenage nephew who was staying with me at the time, was relaxing in a chair close to the piano when the request came for the said racket. He knew at once that it would be a mistake to offer the whole truth, to admit that the warped wooden implement must have been thrown out years before. Instead, he embarked on a pretend search of Farrow Hall and, when that little ruse was beginning to pall, he asked Nakita if she had seen his uncle's tennis racket.

Nakita shot him a contemptuous look.

"What? A tennis racket? Who on earth would want a tennis racket in here?"

James, who had not considered the possible repercussions to his mischief, did his best to put his question into some kind of context.

"I'm only asking because I'm sure I heard someone saying that you were keen on tennis the other day. You mentioned that you played for Kent against Surrey, didn't you?"

With that, he was back in favour and happy to take what he deserved in the form of a three-setter of a story as to how Nakita had won the sixth and last singles in that match and that it had turned out to be the decider. (In short, she had finished things off with a smash, something which was not too difficult to imagine when you considered some of her more brusque comments.)

Norman, by then, had other issues on his mind. He brushed aside all further mentions of a lost racket as the yoga teacher, who came each week, walked through the door hanging on to a bag of balls, light weights and hoops. At that, he hurried to a seat at the back of the room and appeared not to hear the lady's entreaties that he should sit more towards the front of the class.

The yoga, as always, was perhaps the most worthwhile and well-attended activity of the lot at Farrow Hall. Guy Clutterbuck, the old surgeon, kept reiterating that it was very good for them all, while steadfastly refusing to get involved himself. Instead, he came to join Norman and myself for a quiet chat in the corner.

Most of Guy's problems were down to arthritic knees which left him focusing, darkly, on how much longer, if at all, he would be able to walk. Norman evinced a bit of concern regarding his condition, but only insofar as to whether or not he was still able to play football. Guy explained, very reasonably, that his footballing days were long since past and, as Norman drifted off to sleep, so Dorothy's husband, Bernhard, joined the group.

Bernhard who, like his wife, was eighty-three, had forgotten all about the weekly yoga class and walked into the room on tiptoe. He knew only too well that if Dorothy was distracted she would lose all interest in the session.

Dorothy's level of understanding presented problems, with Bernhard never quite knowing how best to explain their situation to her. More often than not, this former judge would admit to being too old and shaky to look after her, a statement which would prompt a terse, two-part retort along the lines that there was nothing wrong with him and that she did not in any case require any help.

Yet on those occasions when Dorothy was safely asleep or out of the way, Bernhard had harrowing tales to tell of how, before she was admitted to Farrow Hall, he only had to nod off in his armchair for five minutes for her to disappear. Other people in their handsome block of flats – Bernhard's brother had designed them 20 years earlier – looked out for her but there had been several occasions when she had slipped out of the building unnoticed and headed for the busy main road and the shops on its far side.

He had imagined that things would be easier when Dorothy was in the care home. Instead, he had found himself faced with a fresh set of worries, not the least of which revolved around the daily pantomime which took place when he would tell her that it was time for him to go home for his supper. At that, she would rise from her chair and protest in a way that surprised residents and visitors alike. Bernhard would try to reason with her in his own gentlemanly way but there were days when he would be trembling with the embarrassment of it all.

On that summer's afternoon, he was enjoying having a chat with people who understood. That was the thing.

Close relatives of the residents and old medical men such as Guy, who were there because of their physical frailty rather than anything else, had plenty in common. They were so much more understanding than those occasional visitors who would airily advise that they had never seen the resident they had come to see looking better. (In other words, they wanted to know why he/she had needed to be in the home in the first place.)

Depending on who that occasional visitor was, you might try to explain about a person with dementia being able to raise his/her game when someone they had not seen in a while paid a visit. But it did not take too many doubtful looks to have you giving up. Regardless of how much it hurt, it was probably easier to let people think what they liked.

Dorothy was usually in good humour after the yoga class but not on this particular occasion. The moment the teacher had said her goodbyes, the old lady was in a state and, for once, it had nothing to do with Bernhard. Her glasses had disappeared.

She said, amid sobs, that she had made sure to put them somewhere safe, only now they were nowhere to be seen. "How am I going to read my book?" she asked, plaintively. (Every week she was among the six-or-so strong group who would pluck books from the assortment which arrived on the local library's equivalent of the care home's tea trolley, though whether or not she read what she chose was debatable.)

She identified Nakita, who had shortly before been putting James in his place about a tennis racket, as someone who might be in the know.

Post-yoga, Nakita was looking benignly on everyone and everything. After listening to Dorothy's concerns, she leapt from her seat and offered to return to where Dorothy had been sitting prior to the class: "I'll go and look down the sides of the seat."

I had been about to chip in with an offer of help but, since Nakita seemed to be on top of the situation, I returned to the piano while keeping a watching brief.

With the gaps down the sides of the chair having revealed nothing beyond a single 20p piece, to which no one laid claim, Nakita came up with an alternative suggestion.

"Have you looked in your handbag, my dear?"

"Yes. It was the first place I looked, actually."

"And have you looked on the windowsill, because I've known you put your spectacles down there before."

Dorothy went off to look and was soon giving us a thumbs-down signal. The same applied when she went to look in the cloakroom opposite the lounge.

Nakita stuck to her task and, if she was beginning to feel anything in the way of irritation, she was managing to keep it firmly under wraps.

"How about your bedroom? That must be worth a look."

"Good idea," said Dorothy. "Thank you, Nakita."

She walked out of the door, but barely had she taken a handful of steps down the corridor than she was back, her premature appearance pushing Nakita over the edge.

"What is it now?"

"I can't find my room."

"Don't be ridiculous. You go there every day."

"It's no good being cross with me. I'm in a muddle and I hate being in a muddle."

"Well, you can leave me out of your muddle," said Nakita, who had picked up her handbag and was on the point of making one of her theatrical exits.

"Aren't you going to stay and help?" asked Dorothy.

"No, I've helped you all I can. I've had enough." Nakita set off but, all of a sudden, she appeared to be having second thoughts about that strike of anger as she looked round the room one more time.

Her voice suddenly soft and hesitant, she addressed Dorothy and those sitting in the immediate vicinity. "I don't suppose any of you have seen my navy scarf anywhere, have you?"

Dorothy spun round. "You're cross with me for being in a muddle but *you're* in a muddle, too."

Now it was Nakita's turn to sob. "You're right. Half the time I don't have a clue what I'm doing."

Ever so gently, Dorothy took Nakita by the hand and together they left the room.

Maybe they were setting out on some kind of joint search. Yet it was just as likely that they, like Norman, would soon have forgotten what they were looking for and normal order would be restored.

It was Alphonso who noticed, later, that Nakita was wearing her scarf and Dorothy was peering through her glasses.

"So everything's turned up, has it?"

Alphonso was still well within hearing distance when Nakita turned to Dorothy. "He's a strange one, that nurse. I don't know about you, Dorothy, but I don't have a clue what he's on about."

Chapter 11: The Great Escape

A Monet-type scenario presented itself on 5 July 2013 as a dozen residents sat by a garden pool dappled with lilies and pretty reeds. The sun was bearing down on the water, while there was just enough breeze to make off with John Huntley's Panama hat and leave it teasingly poised on the water's edge.

Rupert Higgins, the tallest of Farrow Hall's residents at six foot three, had both the reach and the implement – a nicely hooked walking-stick – to save the Panama before it toppled into the pond. With Dorothy advising that he should remember to hang on to his own hat, he all but slipped from his seat while executing a successful if unnerving rescue.

Norman flattered Rupert on his stick skills and asked where he had developed them. Rupert was unhurt, and the rest celebrated with a round of applause.

The ladies were looking a picture in their broad-brimmed sun-hats. Yet had Monet still been around to pick out a candidate for a centre-piece, he would assuredly have opted for Dorothy. She was sitting beneath a hazy blue and pink floppy creation which was a perfect match for her dress. And had he entertained second thoughts, he might have considered Annie Lacey-Hallbright who was adding to the serenity of the occasion by snoozing on a green and white striped swing-seat.

The staff were still in recovery after taking as many as twelve residents out into the garden at the one time and, for a good hour following the flying Panama incident, the afternoon was every bit as peaceful as they deserved. The ladies, along with the only three relatives to have come outside, were keeping tabs on a darting goldfish; John Huntley was reading his copy of *The Scotsman*; Rupert Higgins was basking in his success; Guy Clutterbuck was looking at the sky and Norman was apparently quizzing Marlene, one of the two on-duty helpers, about her daily swim. I, meantime, was playing some barely audible background music which could be heard outside as well as in because the French windows were next to the piano.

Every three tunes or so, I went out into the garden to check on Norman and, on one of those occasions, I noticed Mr Marquis standing in a far corner of the gardens and taking a series of photographs which would surely make it into the next of his decidedly tasteful Farrow Hall brochures. You could imagine people flicking through the pages on behalf of an elderly relative and seeing that colourful scene as the clinching factor.

By three-thirty, everyone, outside and in, would have heard the tea trolley rattling in the distance, which was just as well, for May Simpson and Nakita were beginning to get a bit fidgety and had jointly announced that they were ready for one of "the Wednesday cakes" (usually lemon drizzle or coffee). The two of them rose from their seats and told Marlene that they wanted to go and smarten themselves up before the trolley arrived, which was fair enough. In accord with the home's regulations, Marlene went with them and, with the visitors having left, that left Mabel, her niece, in charge of the remaining ten.

Yet barely five minutes after Marlene had disappeared with May and Nakita, Guy Clutterbuck was getting ready to make a move. He said that the heat was killing him and that he wanted to have his tea indoors.

"Can you hang on a minute, Guy?" asked Mabel. "We'll need to wait until Marlene comes back."

"No," said Guy. "I can't wait till Marlene comes back. Why should I?"

Having risen unsteadily to his feet and assembled the two walking-sticks he needed to take some of the pressure off his ninety-year-old knees, he started shuffling towards the door. Mabel tried to slow his exit and was judging things to a nicety when Marlene, May and Nakita came bustling back. Nakita, I think it was, who knocked into the old specialist, causing him to lose his balance. It was not a complete fall, but enough of one to cause him to shed his hat, his glasses and his composure. May and Nakita were asked to stay in the lounge while Marlene and Mabel sorted him out.

The hat was not a problem after Mabel put it back on his head. But Guy was disturbed, and all the more so when it appeared that his glasses had bounced off into one of the flower-beds lining the path. Marlene sent a message to Jim from the maintenance team and the latter was soon sifting through a thorny yellow rose bush on the path's left flank. That didn't work, but the moment he switched to the flowering shrubs on the other side, he spotted the lenses winking at him from a tangle of branches a good four feet off the ground.

Such was the overall palaver that the nine residents who were still sitting around the pond had by then been left to their own devices for five minutes and possibly ten.

With Guy finally tidied up and delivered to a cool corner in the lounge and Nakita asking if she could wait in the hall for a visitor from the Russian Embassy – he was friendly with one of her distant cousins – Marlene was able to turn her attention to the rest.

As she stepped out of the French doors, she emitted a pained yelp.

"Where, in heaven's name, are they?"

I hurried outside as John Huntley was telling her to calm down.

"It's all right," he said. "They've just gone up the road for a few minutes. Norman said they wouldn't be long. And if you want to know how they left, they went out through the garden gate. Norman asked Robert to bring his height to bear on undoing the bolt at the bottom of the gate's far side. To be honest, Robert undid it so easily that they might as well have put the bolt in the conventional place for all the good that it did. He just bent over double, fiddled around with the bolt for a second or two, and the gate swung open. After that, he and Norman led the way and off they all went. I counted them out, if that's any help, and there were seven."

While Marlene stood there, shaking, I slipped inside to alert Alphonso.

"Now Mrs Mair, are you sure they've gone?"

"Well, no. Not a hundred percent, at least. But that's what John Huntley's saying, and what makes it all the more believable is that the gate's swinging to and fro and there's only two of the residents left. One, of course, is John Huntley and the other is Annie Lacey-Hallbright who's been asleep all afternoon. Apparently, Norman and Rupert led the escapees."

"That figures," said Alphonso.

Alphonso strode into the garden, and from there through the open gate and up to the end of the drive, from which vantage point he glanced up and down the road before shaking his head and coming back to base. His next move was to make a hurried search of the corridors, the garden and the residents' bedrooms before taking up his stance beside a couple of alarm buttons. Five minutes later he pressed the one which would summon Matron and, in this instance, the police.

Matron, who had been off duty for the weekend, usually took ten minutes to get to Farrow Hall from home. On this occasion, she must have made it in three, arriving at precisely the same moment as Mr Marquis came scurrying round the corner with his camera still swinging about his neck and an exasperated look on his face. (News had apparently reached him of Mr Huntley's comments about the poor positioning of the bolt on the gate. It was in fact down to a self-proclaimed nuts and bolts specialist who, after completing a series of tasks at Farrow Hall, had flown off to Australia on the proceeds.)

Nakita, who had picked up on enough snatches of conversation to realise that something or someone had gone missing, started looking behind the curtains and put her Russian visitor in his place when he asked if he should help. "Definitely not," said Nakita. "If anyone notices you lurking behind the curtains, they'll think you're a spy." Guy Clutterbuck, meantime, was crosser than ever, only now it was because no one had brought him his tea. Jennifer Lawrence, a newcomer who had sustained two badly-broken arms when she slipped on her kitchen floor, upset him still further when she said that he should forget about his tea, given the circumstances.

"I'm more worried about the residents," she said, piously, as she and Guy were joined by Alphonso. "You don't," she continued, "think they've been kidnapped, do you?"

Emergency or not, there was the suspicion that Alphonso enjoyed the suggestion.

Alphonso was deployed by Matron to give the police a helping hand with the door-to-door investigation which was about to start in the road outside. Jim, who was a bit miffed at having to stay behind when he should have clocked off from his maintenance tasks twenty minutes earlier, opted to follow Alphonso and I went with him. (At this stage, we were both seeing the supposed emergency as much ado about nothing. There was no way the residents could have gone very far if, indeed, they had gone anywhere. We thought that they would turn up in the back kitchen.)

The two policemen began by knocking on the door of the old grey rectory at the bottom of the hill. The young rector came hurrying out of the house and directed us to the church door with a possibly unwarranted degree of expectation: "I think we're going to find them in here."

The police did not look convinced but were polite enough to agree that it was "a good call". They then watched with interest as the vicar made a production of approaching the church door on tiptoe and opening it so quietly as to suggest he did not want to disturb the missing persons.

In fact, the church was empty bar a couple of ladies doing the flower arranging. They were hurrying to get the place ready for evensong and, as a result, did not welcome the interruption.

The neighbouring homeowners were similarly irked at being disturbed. Although one elderly couple showed willing by following the police out to the road and turning their heads this way and that, the rest shut their doors rather more quickly than they had opened them.

The next port of call was the fish van. It always came on a Wednesday at that hour. The fishmonger wanted to know what all the fuss was about and, when the police complained that Farrow Hall was missing a few residents, he said he knew the feeling. He was missing his usual quota of customers.

Jim and I were on the point of going back to Farrow Hall to look in the kitchen when we spotted a third policeman talking to a woman 50 yards further up the hill. The woman, who was wearing an oversized blue and white striped shirt, possibly a pyjama top, was waving a garden trowel about the place. We joined the rest in hurrying to the scene in time to hear what was clearly the second half of an excruciating exchange.

"I most certainly am not a Farrow Hall resident!"

By then, Alphonso, Jim and I had recognised the woman as Lucy Cavendish, the daughter of a resident. Lucy's mother, Nicola, was the seldom-seen occupant of Room 31 on Farrow Hall's first floor.

Miss Cavendish Junior, as Lucy liked to be known, was a fearsome soul at the best of times and one whose every visit to Farrow Hall involved her producing a leather notebook detailing what her mother should have for her breakfast the following day. Now, she swung round to address the advancing Alphonso. "For your information, Alphonso, I didn't step out on to the road to be abused, which is what's going on here. The reason I came out was to say that your residents aren't lost."

"Thank heavens for that – and thank you, Miss Cavendish." Studiously ignoring her altercation with the policeman, Alphonso asked for the whereabouts of his charges.

"Follow me and I'll show you," she said.

She led Alphonso and Jim, along with the policeman and myself, round the path beside her house whilst explaining how she and her cousin Edna had been tidying up the front garden when they noticed an unlikely-looking crew traipsing up the road.

"I couldn't think who they could be for a minute, and then I recognised Norman from seeing him at Farrow Hall. So I waved and he waved back – and then he led them all across the road. We sort of realised what had happened, and that's when young Edna (young Edna would have been in her sixties) told them, with all her usual presence of mind, that we'd been expecting them.

"So we took them down to the end of the back garden where we'd put seats out for the barbecue we're having tonight for some neighbours. I took down their names in my notebook because I was about to ring you with the details when this policeman appeared.

"Anyhow, here's Edna, now, and there's your residents behind that row of trees to the left."

Edna, as she turned to greet us, was holding an empty plate.

"They've eaten all the sausage rolls," she muttered, "and the one you called Norman has been asking for more, and then he said he would have liked the first lot to have stayed in the oven for a bit longer.

"The cheek of it!" said Lucy Cavendish. Alphonso stifled some laughter while checking that everyone on Lucy's list corresponded with his. He then rang Matron to tell her of the happy outcome and asked if she would send the home's minibus to collect the party.

That done, he thanked Miss Cavendish and her cousin for making his residents so welcome before helping to escort the Farrow Hall Seven to the front of the house to await the driver.

The policeman was the next to inform his superior, "I've found the missing persons, Sir."

He smiled as he fielded what was obviously a compliment.

The combination of that smile and his departure from the truth was all too much for Miss Cavendish. Her face darkened.

"You? You didn't find anyone!"

Alphonso, who was by then safely aboard the minibus himself, pulled the door shut, murmuring that he was not about to get involved.

Miss Cavendish, as it turned out, was dealing with the situation very well on her own.

Jim and I had decided to walk back and, as we turned to wave goodbye to the sisters, we witnessed a fascinating touch of role-reversal. Lucy had brought out that leather notebook of hers and was taking down the policeman's details.

Chapter 12: Hang On to What You've Got

Alan Foster, a retired pharmacist who was married to Maisie, arrived at the piano's side just as I was signing off from that old and much-loved Vera Lynn number, 'We'll Meet Again'.

"That's Maisie's favourite song," he said, by way of opening a conversation. "She used to hum it all the time when she was at home. I'd love it if you'd play it again and then, when you've finished, if you and Norman would join the two of us for a cup of tea. The trolley's on its way and I'm about to tell Maisie something which would have made her very angry on my behalf three or four years ago. It won't mean anything to her at this stage, but it might just be of interest to you."

I watched Maisie as I repeated her favourite song and, even though there was nothing about her face to suggest it meant anything, she was humming the last couple of lines as Alan led the way to where he wanted our little party to sit. He signalled for me to take a chair looking out over the garden while Maisie and Norman sat with their backs to the window.

Alan loved to talk; he missed his former conversations with Maisie, especially when the two of them had had so much in common. Though she, like him, had been a pharmacist before they had a family, her dementia had put paid to the to-ing and fro-ing of meaningful chat, while her lively sense of humour had similarly given up on her. She still made the odd comment to make you wonder whether there was something she found amusing, but it went no further than that.

Alan, a tall, thin figure whose round and heavy spectacles could have been designed for those trying to read prescriptions rather than write them, waited for the tea to be delivered before letting fly with what was indeed a cautionary opening line.

"Whatever else you do, don't let anyone in your family tidy up around you until you're gone."

There was a pause for effect before he explained that his and Maisie's middle daughter, Jane, had raided his bookshelves and told him that she had taken the contents off to some charity shop.

"She waited until I was out at my brother James's place and then she cleared eight shelves' worth of books or, to put it another way, a collection going back fifty years. There were fifty-three editions of Wisden cricket annuals from the 1960s onwards; two rows of books on football and golf, a couple of well-leafed tomes on grammar, thirty of Agatha Christie's novels and so much more.

"She even disposed of a pile of special newspapers that I'd stored since the '60s and, believe it or not, the Wimbledon annual which she herself had given me only a couple of years ago."

There was another pause, this one allowing him to draw breath while simultaneously assimilating further the mischief that had been done to him. Maisie may not have been able to comprehend but her expression was somehow in keeping with his tale of woe.

Then he resumed with the background information.

"Jane said it had to happen, the clearing out, I mean. She said I'd have to downsize soon and there wouldn't be any room for 'my library', as she calls it, in a new place.

"What downsizing, I wanted to know. I told her in no uncertain terms that it didn't need to happen and that it wasn't *going* to happen. I'm happy in my home of fifty-five years and I've always enjoyed the company of my books and papers. They're like old friends."

I felt sorry for this bereft old man whilst sparing a thought for Jane. I remembered how desperate I used to get when Norman would stack box upon box of newspapers in a cellar, turning the house into a veritable tinder box. Occasionally, I would succumb to the temptation to put the odd pile of papers in the bin, but I had learned the hard way that that was never a good idea. At least one of the missing papers would suddenly become the focal point of some frenzied, all-hands-on-deck search the following day.

I admitted the error of my ways to Alan while Norman was speaking to Maisie but, far from tutting, he used my confession as a springboard to his description of how Jane's devious activities had come to light.

"My brother rang me when I had got home from the visit I was telling you about. He wanted me to look up my copy of the 1962 Wisden guide to see if Richie Benaud had played in the Australian side that won the Ashes, or whether he was a non-playing captain. Now I didn't need to look it up because I knew that Benaud had been injured, but I always like to double-check. So I told James to hang on a minute while I went to look – and what did I find but a near-empty bookcase? All I could see were a couple of cookery books which had belonged to Maisie rather than me."

As Alan paused again, I seized the opportunity to ask if Jane was even vaguely interested in sport.

He laughed heartily at that. "Is Jane interested in sport? Heavens no! She's always been a workaholic, a true academic who steadfastly refuses to waste her time *playing* anything. Economics was – and still is – her thing. I tried to get her interested in golf a few years ago but she didn't approve of the way women had to play second fiddle to the men at the club. Can't say I blame her, but she stirred up so much trouble that I was mighty relieved when she said she never wanted to hit another ball. To be honest, I got the impression that the members of the committee were furious with me for having brought her along in the first place.

"Funnily enough," he continued, and there was no stopping him now, "Jane's sisters and their brother, Eddie, have always been quite the opposite. Eddie, in particular, refused to waste his time working when he could be chasing a ball. To be fair to Jane, though, I get the feeling that she's been a bit bored since she retired from her job in the City, and moved back to Scotland. I may be wrong, but I'm pretty sure that that's what's behind this bout of interference."

Alan's dilemma had been overheard by Dorothy's husband Bernhard and, as Dorothy was half-asleep, he had wandered across to join our group, his stoop and general stiffness more discernible than ever.

"I hope you don't mind me coming over like this," he said, "but I heard some of what you were saying and it struck a chord. My daughter Sally took a whole pile of my clothes down to the charity shop in Peebles not so long ago and, like your Jane, she didn't even ask. Damn nuisance these daughters."

"You can say that again," chuckled Alan. Norman concurred.

Bernhard endeavoured to stretch to his full height, the better to show off the tweed jacket which was about to get a mention.

"This was just one of the items she snapped up," he said. "Dorothy had gone to the lengths of getting some leather patches sewn on to the elbows four or five years ago and it's been as good as new ever since; it remains my favourite jacket by miles. We'd bought the tweed when we were visiting a place called Bunabhainneadar – I'm probably not pronouncing it right – on the West coast of the Isle of Harris. It wasn't really a shop, more a barrow on the driveway up to the little croft where the cloth had been woven."

"I'd love to know how you got the jacket back," said Alan and, if he sounded a bit impatient, which I thought he did, you had to suspect that he was worried lest Bernhard was about to embark on the finer details of the tweed's background and that his own story might be overtaken.

Bernhard got the message.

"The moment I realised what had happened, I drove down to Smythson's, a charity shop in Peebles which the family had visited for years. It's quite famous, you know. Anyhow, after a quick look round the old clothes department, I spotted my jacket and six or seven of my sweaters on a rail of their own. There was a lady labelling them and I interrupted her to say that the moment she'd finished, I would buy the lot.

"She looked at me in utter astonishment before saying that at the very least I should try on the jacket.

"So I told her I didn't need to try it on because I'd been wearing it for the last quarter of a century."

Even Alan was tickled by a tale which offered such hope. From that point, there was not so much as a hint of hastiness in his voice and general demeanour. Rather was he listening intently, maybe in the hope of picking up a few tips.

Apparently, the woman had called for the manageress, who in turn said that he could have everything back for nothing more than a £10 service charge. Of course, the two women wanted to know what had happened and, when he told them that it was down to one of his daughters who had decided that he had too much clutter, they said that it was usually a daughter who wrought that kind of havoc. Wives, apparently, seldom had the guts to go through with it.

A couple of weeks later, when Alan's and my paths crossed in the Farrow Hall entrance, I seized the opportunity to ask if he had had any luck in retrieving his books.

He was excited to be the bearer of good news.

"They're all back in their rightful places, thank you very much."

I asked if he had gone down the Smythson's route and he shook his head. That had been his intention, only it hadn't been necessary.

When word had spread among family members of what Jane had done, each of her siblings had given her a rocket and, as she was relieved to be able to report, the books had gone no further than the back of her car.

"She returned them to my shelves only two days after we had that conversation over tea," said Alan. Not only that, but the dear girl added a note of apology which was attached to a nicely-wrapped present – a copy of the latest Wisden annual."

Chapter 13: Yellow Dusters

Annie Lacey-Hallbright, who was a resident in Farrow Hall more because she was worried about what the future held than anything else, was what you might call a volunteer helper. Belinda McDonald, on the other hand, was a sixty-nine-year-old dementia victim who saw herself as a member of staff.

To the uninitiated at least, it seemed that she was a victim of what they call OCD or Obsessive Compulsive Disorder. In her case, it manifested itself in a passion for housework which had started when she lived in her own home. In itself, it was harmless enough, but over time she had developed some altogether more worrying traits which included leaving the doors wide open at night, a situation which was not lost on a couple of young thieves walking back from a nearby pub one evening. They made off with a couple of bags of the family silver.

When the time came for Belinda to move to Farrow Hall, she brought her own supply of dusters and polish and, no doubt wisely, the staff hurriedly substituted a couple of plastic pots of innocuous polish – it said on the label that it was for children's dolls' houses – for her potentially more toxic supermarket variety.

I had heard a lot about the lady, but she was not someone we knew well on the ground floor. She occupied Room 17 on the first floor and took her meals in the first-floor dining room. In keeping with which, all her polishing of doorknobs and window-sills took place along the upstairs corridors and she expressed no interest in covering new ground. That is, until Betsy, with her ballroom dancing background and love for any kind of musical get-together, suggested they go down together for a Tuesday piano session.

The dusters, most of them in that traditional sunflower yellow, came with them and, almost before I had finished playing that afternoon, Belinda was dusting the piano legs. When Norman told her to put her dusters away, she gave him a black look.

Matron, who had heard Norman's terse instruction, quickly went to great lengths to speak to the people seated around the piano about how much she admired

Belinda's work. "This is kind of Belinda, don't you think? I keep telling her that she doesn't need to do it but that's not what she wants to hear."

"I couldn't be happier," said Belinda. "Everyone appreciates what I do and I'm not going to let them down. Only this morning, Major Briggs, that nice man who's staying here while his housekeeper is away, said that I make a better job of the brass doorknobs than any of the privates in his regiment. He says he'd trust me to clean anything."

"Be careful!" laughed Alphonso, who had joined us. "If I know the Major, he'll be telling you to clean his shoes before you know where you are."

Belinda answered with a doubtful chuckle which continued to reverberate as she set off on a working trip of the very different labyrinth of corridors which lay outside the downstairs lounge. More sills, more brass doorknobs.

You could not fail to notice that Belinda had much the same well-polished air as everything she touched. Her puffs of white hair floated above a shiny weather-beaten face, while her clothes were usually navy and always spotless. In fact, all her outfits were washed and pressed by a personal laundry service operated by her older sister, Maria. As Maria said to me one afternoon, Belinda always looked as if she was going out for the day as opposed to busying herself with some mundane housework.

Belinda and Betsy had disappeared and I was about to pack up for the evening when Annie alerted me to the fact that a handful of dusters were still lying under the piano.

I gathered them up in the hope of catching up with their owner; only by the time I looked out into the corridor, I realised that time was of the essence. Belinda was on her own down at the far end of the main corridor and about to take a left turn towards what was generally seen as Professor Perkins's jigsaw territory. Professor Perkins, who had her jigsaw laid out in an area where the corridor expanded to accommodate a large bay window, would not be pleased to see her. However, just as I was well on my way to catching her, Annie called after me to say that I'd dropped a couple of dusters on the way.

By the time I had retraced my footsteps and picked them up, the inevitable was happening. Belinda was getting it in the neck from Dr Perkins.

"I want your name; your full name, if you don't mind."

"Belinda McDonald."

"Well, Belinda. It seems that no one has told you what's what in this part of Farrow Hall. I'm afraid you've broken the rules already."

The best I could do at this point, for I was as wary of Professor Perkins as anyone else, was to stand by whilst trying to lighten the mood with a smile.

"What rules?" asked Belinda. "I was only going to polish the desk."

Professor Perkins waved her hands by way of drawing an imaginary line across that area where the corridor coincided with her annex.

"See this line," she began.

"What line?" said Belinda.

"If you pay attention, you'll see that I'm showing you the join in the carpet which indicates where my territory begins and yours ends. If you keep to your side of the line, there won't be a problem. I'll let you step on to my side of the line when I've finished my jigsaw, which should be in approximately two weeks' time." (Belinda would not have known that the jigsaw was something of an unfinished symphony in that Dr

Perkins would remove two handfuls of pieces last thing every evening, usually with her eyes shut, and put them in one of the drawers below.)

A baffled Belinda agreed to conform and, as the two of us made our way back to the lounge, she regaled a couple of sister members of the cleaning corps with details of the curious happenings. Both women agreed that she had plenty to do without going near the jigsaw lady. In fact, they had another job she might like.

They asked her to tend the granite work surface above the dining-room units, the area from which morning coffees and afternoon teas were usually dispensed.

To Belinda, this was the ultimate honour. The work surface was a dazzling black and sea-blue granite, and doorknobs and sills were forgotten as she polished it over and over. It made you think of those brave men who, in days gone by, would get to the end of painting the old Forth Railway Bridge, only to return to the beginning and start again.

Matron always made a point of congratulating Belinda on her work and, when Maria came on her twice-weekly visit, she would check that the sister was happy with the routine Belinda had adopted for herself.

"It's the best thing that could have happened," said Maria. "She's never been able to sit still and it would be a sin to try and make her. She's happier here than she's been in years and it's a lot to do with the cleaning. I'll tell you how it all started, if you like, though it's a long story."

"I could do with one of those," said Connie as she collapsed into a nearby chair. "I've been on my feet all day. Mind you, don't make it too long because I'm interviewing a new care worker in half an hour."

"That's fine," said Maria. "I'll just skip mentioning a couple of her cleaners.

"Belinda," she began, "used to live with her husband Peter in an old stone house in the Grange area of Edinburgh. Peter was a headmaster and she was head of house in the same school.

"They had everything they wanted, including a really excellent cleaner. Annabel might have been in her seventies but she was still brilliant, so it was such a shame when she died. What's more, Peter died the very same week. Can you believe it? Heart attacks, both of them."

Connie and I nodded in sympathy. "What a terrible thing to happen," said Connie.

"Belinda didn't know what had hit her. She just couldn't cope. I realised that the best thing would be to find her a new cleaner, but the first one I got was a disaster. Total disaster. Joanne had come courtesy of a local agency but she spent more time making coffee for herself – it had to be the real stuff too! – than doing any work. The agency said they were ever so sorry and sent over another girl, Marianne. Now, she could clean, but she also needed to have her radio on all the time. Belinda took refuge in the garden whenever she was there; only when she came in there was never any sign that Marianne had done much to earn her keep."

By now Maria was counting cleaners on her fingers and, having described two, she cut out numbers three and four.

"Number five left of her own accord: she said the job was too much for her. She was followed by a girl called Sue who came via a friend of a friend. Belinda liked her a lot but still there was something wrong.

"I had been noticing a difference in my sister's behaviour by then. She had started washing her hands every few minutes and, the moment Sue arrived, she would start to follow the poor girl around the house.

"Sue spoke to me about it and between us we decided that Belinda needed to see her doctor. The latter suspected the beginnings of dementia.

"When Sue left because she could take no more, Belinda did her own cleaning and I have to say she could not have made a better job of it. But the cleaning was getting more and more obsessive, as was everything else about her behaviour. Most of the peculiar happenings were harmless enough; only then she stopped locking up in the evenings and these young lads got in through the kitchen door and made off with a bunch of Waitrose bags, all of them full of silver. Neighbours rang for the police and, though all the stolen goods were returned – at least we hoped it was all of them – that was the first step towards Belinda's road to Farrow Hall."

Matron thanked Maria for her account and said that it was always good to hear more about a resident's background.

Maria thanked her for listening and was heading out of the room when she came to a sudden halt.

"I know this sounds a bit crazy," she said, "but Belinda's told me a couple of times now that she'd like the same blue overalls as the other ladies wear on cleaning duty. I don't mind paying for it, but is that possible?"

Matron was used to getting some oddball requests but this was the strangest yet.

She called Alphonso across; he, inevitably, was all in favour.

He sent Janice, who helped out in the laundry from time to time, to fetch a fresh overall and everyone in the room was encouraged to applaud as Matron announced that Belinda had been made an honorary member of the cleaning corps.

Later in the day, Alphonso asked me what I thought of the arrangement. I said I loved the way Farrow Hall gave their residents a free rein, whenever that was possible.

Only the week before, they had accommodated Norman when he insisted on attending a meeting of the Farrow Hall Board and staff members. According to Alphonso, they had already taken their places when Norman arrived and noticed a vacant seat next to Sir Rodney Allen, the chairman. Norman assumed it was for him and Alphonso had a word with Matron, who agreed that it would be easier to let him stay.

There had been no sign of Norman, either in the lounge or in his room, when I had arrived at Farrow Hall that day but, when I heard voices coming from the now closed-off dining room area, I had a quick peep through the crack in the double doors – and there he was. He was sitting alongside all the other attendees, with a folder of information in front of him.

I continued to keep half an eye on proceedings as the meeting was drawing to a close with the usual Any Other Business. That was when Norman stood up and said that as far as he knew, there had been no fresh supply of rugby balls.

Alphonso took charge.

"Thank you for that, Norman," he said. "I'm making a note of what you're saying and will try and get it sorted out."

"Quite," said Sir Rodney, with an emphatic nod of the head.

Alphonso could always be relied upon to come up with a comment to suit the moment. And when, as the meeting closed, Norman said he was catching the bus into town, Alphonso put a stop to that with an entirely plausible story: the bus drivers had gone on strike as from midday.

But the situation which arose the following week was hardly one for which Alphonso had an explanation to hand.

The usual crowd of Nakita, Dorothy, Alicia and Annie had expanded. Major Briggs, Mr Huntley and May Simpson had joined them for the piano session and they were all were enjoying that 'Yi Yi Yipee Yipee Yi' chorus, when something caught my eye.

A shoe flew past the lounge window, and then another and another.

I alerted Alphonso to what I thought was happening at the same time as Dorothy backed up my story.

"I've just seen shoes falling from the sky," said Dorothy.

"Don't be ridiculous," countered Nakita. "Pigs may fly but shoes don't."

"What's all that about, Nakita?" asked Matron.

"Dorothy's being ridiculous. She said she saw shoes flying past the window."

By then, Alphonso was beginning to have his suspicions. He tore upstairs and five minutes later returned to the room with his arm around an emotional Belinda.

Even before they pulled up, Belinda was offering an explanation.

"You know what Alphonso said the other day about how Major Briggs would soon be telling me to clean his shoes? Well, he handed me two pairs this morning and asked me to get them done by lunchtime because he had relatives coming for tea. He said he hadn't decided which pair he would be wearing at that point, so I was to do both.

"I'd always liked the man up until then but, when I told him that I wasn't going to get my new overall plastered with his beastly black shoe polish, he told me he'd make sure that my honorary cleaner role was stopped straight away.

"He left his shoes outside the door just the same, and that's why I chucked them out of the window."

"Very good," said Alphonso.

Matron gave him a look before turning back to Belinda. "First things first, Belinda. I can assure you that no one is going to take away your title."

Before she moved on to whatever else might have been of note, the Major shot out of the room, saying that he would be back in a trice.

On his return, he made a very public apology.

"I'm afraid I overstepped the mark. I must have thought I was back in the army I'm afraid; it happens to me a lot and I would be very happy if you, Belinda, would accept my apologies, along with this small gift."

He handed over a silver medal which, as he would later reveal, he had been awarded for his role in the organisation of Princess Alice's funeral in 1969. "This," he said, "needs an owner who knows how to keep it shiny."

Belinda uttered a series of 'Thank-yous' before offering to go and collect his shoes from the flower-bed.

"Definitely not," said Major Briggs. "It would be a travesty if I didn't go outside and pick them up for myself."

Chapter 14: Puzzling

Professor Margaret Mary Perkins, who had a medical background, was proud of being over a hundred, only she was not entirely sure how much over. "I could be 103, but one of my daughters says I'm 104. I'm inclined not to believe her because she's in her late 70s and has never been any good at facts and figures." The professor said that she kept meaning to ask Matron to come up with the answer but had decided against the idea after thinking that everyone in the home might start expecting the staff to look into such trivia when they should be dealing with more important issues.

What bothered her rather more was that she was confined to a wheelchair. She could still struggle about her bedroom by holding a walking-stick in one hand and leaning on the furniture with the other, only that no longer worked when it came to venturing outside her door.

There was something else which irked her, too. Though the staff at the home would come running when she summoned them with two sharp rings of her bell, she did not always get the immediate follow-on attention she felt she deserved. She had to wait her turn.

Every morning, Professor Perkins liked to be wheeled to this small annex off one of the corridors, an area over which, as Belinda had discovered to her cost, she had somehow managed to convey ownership. There was a desk which had originally been seen as somewhere a resident might go to write a good old-fashioned letter to her relatives, but Professor Perkins would tell her fellow residents that her thousand-piece jigsaw puzzle of Edinburgh took precedence over any letter writing. As for a recent arrival who came to her neck of the woods bearing a jigsaw of his own, he was told to set up shop in Farrow Hall's back porch because it was her jigsaw which visitors expected to see. According to the lady herself, he disappeared without further ado.

Visitors who did arrive on the professor's patch were given a lengthy lecture on how an earlier edition of her Edinburgh jigsaw boasted neither a bypass, a modern tram network, a Harvey Nichols, or even the parliament building at Holyrood, of which she did not approve.

The professor could access all corners of the city from her wheelchair while keeping herself snug under a MacGregor tartan rug, a handsome item which had been given to her by the parishioners at the local Episcopal Church. Her clothes usually included one tartan or another but, by way of a constant, her hair was arranged in a handsome if hurriedly assembled bun. According to Alphonso, she would become quite agitated if anyone fussed over stray strands. Her argument was that at her age, whatever it was, she hardly had time to be bothered with such minutiae and that it was more important to her that the pieces of her jigsaw should be in their rightful places.

It was on an October day in 2013 that the professor was presiding over her puzzle when my twin granddaughters who, having done the rounds of all the residents, went along to see how she was progressing. The pair began by watching from a distance of around 30 yards but, before too long, they were inveigled into getting down on their hands and knees to peer under the desk for one among the thousand pieces. Just in case it helped, the old lady told them she thought it was part of the Scott Monument on Princes Street. The girls found it and, by way of a reward, she let them insert it.

Perhaps it was because they had made such a worthwhile contribution that Professor Perkins was prompted to launch into a complaint about her son, Mark. He always had an excuse as to why he could not appear when she needed him and, that very morning, he had been particularly perverse. When she rang to ask if he would retrieve one of her tweed skirts from a trunk in the family home's attic, he said he was "too tired" to scale the attic steps.

The twins, who seemed to think of a trip into an attic as an exciting mission for anyone's son or daughter, offered to do the job themselves before hurrying back to the lounge to give me an update. (It was probably no coincidence that they arrived hard on the heels of a care worker bearing a chocolate cake.)

As they hurtled towards the piano, Alphonso called across to ask if the professor had been pleased to see them. They nodded enthusiastically and said they would be going back after tea if their grandfather was still asleep.

Alphonso looked doubtful and, once the pair had tucked into some cake and shot off in another direction, he said that it was a miracle that the old lady had put up with them at all. Rumour had it that in her former life as a GP, she had been known to prescribe a particularly foul-tasting castor oil to children who made a nuisance of themselves.

He pointed to a gentleman in the corner who mostly kept himself to himself. "John Huntley, who's sitting over there, was one of her old patients. When they met a month or so ago it was for the first time in sixty years and the poor man was so shell-shocked as to make a mistake for which he is unlikely to be forgiven. He asked after her cat, Clarence, who died in the 1940s.

"Ever since, they have each avoided each other like the plague. On the rare occasions that Professor Perkins sits in the lounge, she'll peep out from over the top of her copy of *The Times* and, if there's any sign of him, she will hide behind it. I think she's terrified that he'll come over and bring her up to speed with his childhood coughs and snivels."

John Huntley's eyes had opened at the mention of his name and, as one of three residents nursing an assortment of broken bones, he hobbled across.

"Did you call me?" he asked.

Alphonso's eyes were full of mischief.

"Not exactly, but I was just mentioning that you used to be one of Professor Perkins's patients."

As Alphonso anticipated, John Huntley seized the opportunity to tell of his never-to-be-forgotten visits to the surgery at No. 2, The Avenue, in Livingston. Ever so slowly, he subsided into a handsome armchair within chatting distance of Norman's seat and the piano stool. He laid his walking-stick down on the floor before lifting his broken leg onto a leather footstool while announcing that he was going to begin at the beginning: in the waiting room.

"I'll grant you," he said, "that there was a roaring fire, but I don't think that it was ever stoked with the patients in mind. It would have been nice if that had been the case, but I know for a fact that it wasn't. It was for the doctor's ancient Uncle Tom and a fat ginger cat called Clarence. Both sat tight in the prime seats and rarely budged."

He recalled an afternoon when a patient with a heart condition shooed Clarence from her chair.

"At that very moment, the doctor burst into the room and made plain that neither Clarence nor the uncle was to be disturbed. And just in case you're interested to know what happened next, the cat gave a knowing look and returned to its seat and my mother gave her chair to the patient with the heart condition. I stayed put on the floor doing the one and only waiting-room jigsaw. The choice was between a jigsaw with more pieces missing than not and an out-of-date copy of the *Illustrated London News*."

John Huntley said he would have loved to have made friends with that cat, only the one time he tried to stroke it he was on the receiving end of a nasty nip which he was stupid enough to report to the doctor. She, in turn, demonstrated her annoyance by picking up a silver tankard of pens and pencils and slamming it down on the desk before announcing that he had been asking for trouble.

It seemed that Mr Huntley blamed his mother more than anyone else for the lady's avid dislike of him. "Heaven knows why, but my mother would drag me along to see her at the first sign of a cough or sneeze. And every time I went into that darned surgery, I would come out feeling worse than when I went in because all the windows were wide open, with the net curtains billowing like sails at sea. The usual routine was that my teeth would start to chatter and she would prescribe two teaspoons of castor oil a day from one of those sticky brown bottles. I'm pretty sure that the size of the dose was to discourage me from coming back, only my mother wouldn't hear of it. She said that the doctor was very conscientious and that the visits were necessary, 'just to be on the safe side'."

Mr Huntley was not about to claim that his mother and the doctor had done him any lasting harm in that he was seventy-nine and his only complaint was temporary: the broken leg and wrist he had sustained when he tumbled ten feet from one layer of his prize vegetable patch onto the rockery below. The broken bones may have left him shocked and shaken but, in all honesty, he looked no older than his mid-60s.

His story told, Mr Huntley made a slow and shaky rise from his seat to mark a change of subject.

"You know what, it's time for me to stop talking and for you to play the piano. Whenever I tell my Professor Perkins story, I'm reminded of an old record which the uncle used to play over and over, one where the chorus began with the line, '*Ten cents a dance, that's what they pay me.*' You can't play it by any chance, can you?"

Against all the odds, I could. It was the penultimate number on a disc I had picked up in a second-hand bookshop on the way into town a couple of weeks earlier. I hadn't heard anything particularly catchy in the first ten or so tunes and had been about to turn to the radio when the 'Ten cents a dance' number came up. I stayed with it because I rather liked its sad sway.

Mr Huntley was intrigued to hear it again, and went on to ask if I knew various other tunes from the same era. When it was all getting a bit embarrassing as I admitted to knowing no more than one in five, I excused myself on the grounds that I needed to check up on the twins.

Jessica and Charlotte had repaired to the professor's eyrie and, just as I turned a corner in the corridor which gave me a view, there was a pained cry from the old lady as Edinburgh's south-west region, bypass and all, toppled in slow motion to the floor. Some pieces had taken off individually, others in parties of five or six, with each piece of the larger groups clinging to the others for dear life. Charlotte was a ghostly white.

To my utter astonishment, the professor took this disaster in her stride. The initial shock over, she mentioned that she had lived through the Blitz before adding that she, rather than Charlotte, was to blame. "I made the mistake of moving the puzzle to the point where it was hanging over the front edge of the desk. My apologies."

There was more potential for trouble when the girls tried to jam a few pieces from the ruins of Lauriston Castle into a modern housing scheme but, here again, the three sorted things out amicably enough and the professor confided that when it came to jigsaws the two of them were in a different league to Mark.

The mention of Mark reminded the girls that she had previously described her son's refusal to go into the attic to fetch her skirt. Jessica restarted the conversation by asking how old Mark was.

There was a pause before the doctor dropped something of a bombshell.

"He's seventy-five."

The girls struggled to digest that piece of information. "He's *what*?"

Professor Perkins enjoyed their bewilderment. Then she upped the decibels, as if to deliver the information not just to everyone in Farrow Hall but the entire neighbourhood: "I said my son's SEVENTY-FIVE!"

The repetition prompted a spate of uneasy giggles and, after I had given hasty consideration to what Alphonso and Mr Huntley had been saying about the lady's dislike of irritating children, I stepped forward to whisk them away.

Charlotte had other ideas. She had one more question she 'had' to ask. She wanted to know if Professor Perkins ever wished she was still a doctor.

When she replied, "Every now and then I do," I sensed what was coming next. Charlotte held aloft the left-hand finger she had shut in the car door the previous day and asked if she would take a look. And Jessica, not to be outdone, hurriedly chimed in with the thought that she might want to examine her tonsils.

Professor Perkins straightened herself up and went to work.

Jessica, with her tonsillitis, was summoned first.

"Open your mouth and say, 'Aaaaah!!' if you don't mind," said the professor. By way of a bit of make-believe, she used her heavily finger-printed monocle to feign a serious stare into the abyss.

"In my day," she continued, "some doctors would have said that you might need to have those tonsils out at some point. I never went along with all that nonsense and, from what I can see, your tonsils can stay put."

Then she called for the injured finger to be held up again: "You need to keep moving it around like this, you see, and it'll be all right before you know it."

There was never any mention of castor oil, nor did she tell them to run along. Instead, in what John Huntley would no doubt have called an extraordinary turn of events, she patted them on the head and suggested a return visit in a couple of days.

Chapter 15: The Christmas Party

There was no need for another Christmas party when there were already more than enough activities on Farrow Hall's Christmas agenda and had been since early November. But, with a handsome tree standing in one corner of the lounge, and plenty of decorations to capture the festive spirit, the residents were some way removed from greeting the latest fixture with a weary sigh.

Carol singers had already come from each of the churches and primary schools in the area, along with other organisations such as the local book club and the Ramblers' Association. Two high school choirs were due, as was the Salvation Army and a gathering of Army wives. Yet, rightly or wrongly, I thought there was room for Farrow Hall to stage its own concert in amongst the rest. My idea was that the residents would dictate the content.

When Alphonso and I agreed on 18 December as an appropriate date, my first move was to type out a list of carols from which the residents could make their choices. I printed off enough sheets for everyone and handed them round ahead of afternoon tea at the start of the month.

You would not think that a carol concert in a care home would make for trouble, what with the emphasis on Peace on Earth and Goodwill to Men, etc., but all that was lost on Nakita. She studied the list of carols for a moment before laying it down in an emphatic and angry fashion.

"If you don't mind," she said, "I'm not going to waste my time on any of this nonsense because I'm about to turn on the television."

Annie Lacey-Hallbright, who usually steered clear of any impending row, spoke out at once: "Excuse me, Nakita, but that won't do. If someone's been kind enough to ask us to choose the carols, that's what needs to happen."

Alicia, another who normally contrived to steer well clear of Nakita, took Annie's side in the argument. "You've done this kind of thing before, 'Madame'

Nakita. Go and watch the television in your own room and let the rest of us get on with the job."

Nakita did not budge; she sat there and she simmered. Others, meantime, were ready with their suggestions, with the first contribution coming from Dorothy.

"I don't think we should begin with this one, but I'd like to vote for 'Ding Dong Merrily on High'. It's a splendid old carol, especially when it's well sung."

Norman said he did not give a damn who sung what as long as he did not have to join in, and next up was John Huntley who had stayed at Farrow Hall for longer than anticipated after his broken bones had to be reset. He asked for 'We Three Kings' on the grounds that he had been a king – he had been trusted with the phial of myrrh – in a school nativity play sixty-five years before.

We were up to six carols by the time Nakita had recovered sufficiently from the reprimands to make her own submission.

"I'd like to choose one, if you don't mind, though I have to say it's a great pity that you didn't ask me first. I sang in the Perth choir until I was in my late fifties and I know how these things work."

Annie and not a few others raised their eyebrows.

"I'd like 'Hark the Herald Angels Sing'," continued Nakita. "It's a wonderful carol and, if you're worried about the refrain, I will be able to help out. I'm good on the high notes. In fact, I used to sing the whole thing as a solo, in Russian would you believe, and could do the same again if required."

My intervention was a spur-of-the-moment affair. I told Nakita that I was sure she would have sung it beautifully but that we had a rather different task in mind for her. My impromptu thought was that she could present a bouquet to the grandmother of the soloist.

Nakita smiled a disconcertingly sweet smile at the suggestion. Annie gave a knowing look and, much to my relief, the arrival of afternoon tea and a handful of relatives put the kibosh on any further concerns for the time being.

Annie came over as I was storing my list of carols inside the lid of the piano stool. "Can you tell me the name of the soloist?" she asked.

"Certainly. I think you probably know the girl's grandmother, Mrs Elsie McFee. She lives in the row of cottages where you sometimes go to play cards on a Tuesday evening. I think I heard Alphonso say that you partner her at bridge." (The cottages to which I had referred had been built for local people in the 1880s when money was tight and there were no old age pensions and no National Health Service. Originally, there had been just a handful of homes but, over the next century, they turned the land into a 20-strong development and as pretty a complex as you might find in the south of France. Those lucky enough to acquire a south-facing property always had a handsome array of flowers sitting in the tubs on their front porches.)

Annie knew the granny well and had for long been an avid admirer of her all-year-round floral displays. She also knew Elizabeth, the granddaughter, for the girl would often put her head round the corner of the lounge during the bridge sessions to let her granny know she had arrived. "Has anyone told you," advised Annie, "that Elizabeth is training to be an opera singer at the Royal Conservatoire of Music in Glasgow?"

"No, I hadn't heard that, but how wonderful."

Elizabeth combined her next visit to her grandmother with one to Farrow Hall. She was seventeen years old, had a wonderful crop of golden curls hanging loosely about her shoulders and she was an imposing six feet tall.

An old friend of mine had recommended her and, to my great glee, she was thrilled to be the recipient of our humble invitation. She asked if anyone would mind if her granny came along too. "I'd love her to hear me singing somewhere other than in her own front room," she said. "She doesn't like going out very far nowadays but she's not going to mind the walk to Farrow Hall as it's barely 200 yards."

She said that the two of them would be there from the start to the finish and that her idea for a solo was 'Ave Maria'. As luck would have it, she preferred to sing it without any kind of accompaniment. (My reading of music was never going to be good enough to complement singing of her calibre.)

The big day came.

With the concert due to begin at six thirty, residents had been given an early supper. The staff had set the chairs in a nice curve which would allow for Elizabeth to be the focal point as she sang her solo in front of the Christmas tree.

The residents and their visitors were shown into the room first, shortly to be followed by other visitors. Next, those residents who were wheelchair bound –

there were four of them – were delivered to the front row, either by Alphonso or their visitors.

Professor Perkins, from among the wheelchair contingent, said she was not happy with the arrangements. She wanted to be by the door because she said she would be leaving early. Alphonso said that that was not a good idea: "There's a real treat at the end so I'd stay put if I were you."

Everyone was handed a programme which had a picture of Elizabeth on the cover along with details of her career. The lyrics of the carols followed.

When everything was set, Elizabeth and her granny were escorted into the room by John Marquis and everyone clapped expectantly.

The granny was resplendent in a blue silk dress with silver buttons down the front. As for Elizabeth, she wore a darker shade of blue, almost navy, with black patent high heels and a matching handbag. Had she been singing at the Royal Festival Hall she could not have taken more trouble with her appearance.

"For our first carol," said Mr Marquis, when he had delivered all the usual pleasantries that belong in an introduction, "we're going to have 'We Three Kings,' chosen by John Huntley." John Huntley gave a proud bow at the mention of his name and, though Norman decided to leave midway through the first verse and elbowed aside the nurse who tried to persuade him against the idea, the concert was off to a pretty good start.

When John Marquis announced: "Now we are moving on to 'Hark the Herald Angels Sing', chosen by Nakita," Nakita stood up and held her carol sheet high in front of her.

Alphonso told her to sit down and, to all round relief, she sat.

'Away in a Manger' came next, followed by 'Ding Dong Merrily on High' and 'The First Nowell', with the latter reduced to two verses on account of the raising strains of 'Nowell, Nowell' becoming wincingly out of hand. 'See Amid the Winter's Snow' offered a recovery period, and then it was time for the interval and for the guests to walk about while they were treated to cartons of apple juice provided by the local Tesco store. The audience were enjoying themselves thoroughly, only they couldn't wait to hear Elizabeth.

The plan was that as soon as 'Silent Night' was over, our appointed lighting engineer – my son, Patrick – would turn off the lights as the soloist took up her position, candle in hand. Alas, our engineer had failed to apprise himself of the position of the light switches. Alphonso and the twins stepped in to help, all of which resulted in around five different switches being turned on and off in a spectacle that put one in mind of the Hogmanay firework display from Edinburgh Castle.

At last, the room went dark and Elizabeth stepped out with the candle-light playing on those golden curls.

The teenager sang so sweetly that everyone was spellbound, and no one more so than her granny, whose face glowed only marginally less than the candle.

Elizabeth was inspired. People were shaking their heads in admiration and the girl's confidence was growing by the second.

The first two verses over, she was expanding, quite beautifully, on the 'Mari-i-i-a' which followed the 'Ave' at the start of the third verse when trouble struck. Professor Perkins was the culprit. Straightening herself up in her wheelchair, she emitted a seismic yelp for help: "I've had enough of this!"

"Shut up!" said Nakita.

Elizabeth ignored the goings-on. I could only assume that she had been reared on that old cliché about the show having to go on as she clung heroically to her note during the shenanigans, before slipping seamlessly into the rest of the verse.

With Professor Perkins having been removed, the audience was able to relax and when, finally, things came to a halt, our soloist smiled a slightly embarrassed smile as everyone clapped and cheered.

Though the granny was heard to mutter, "I'd like to get my hands on that Professor Perkins," she said later that the interruption had demonstrated beyond doubt that her granddaughter was made of the right stuff.

Matron came forward to give a vote of thanks and to present Elizabeth with a bouquet, which was graciously received and paved the way for another clapping session.

"And I think," added Matron, "we have something for Elizabeth's granny and I'd be grateful, Mrs McFee, if you'd be good enough to join us on the stage."

Elizabeth made room for her granny, while Nakita, who was wearing a pretty pink sweater for the occasion, acted as primed, picking up a bouquet from under her chair and making her move.

Only instead of stepping on to the stage and making her presentation, she hot-footed it out of the room.

"I think you've forgotten something, Nakita," called a smiling Alphonso. What that something was suddenly clicked with Nakita. She came to a full stop and, *mirabile dictu,* she allowed Alphonso to lead her back on to the stage where she combined her curtsy with an unlikely but thoroughly endearing apology.

Chapter 16: Who is Wearing What

Alphonso looked exasperated. "Mrs Mair," he began, "do you have any idea how long it takes to get them all looking like this?"

Farrow Hall's sage-cum-humorist was reacting to a casual comment I'd made about the residents looking particularly smart that day.

To be honest, I had never given a thought to how long it might take for the staff to get them all dressed in the mornings. The nearest experience on which I could draw revolved around Norman's exploits in the months before he entered the home. He would get up three or four times in the middle of the night and ask for his golf clubs, his gun, or something else pretty random, and the business of persuading him to get undressed and go back to bed never got any easier.

Alphonso gave me a few details about the morning craziness.

"There are plenty of residents who can get themselves ready on their own, as long as they don't have too many physical challenges. But it's very different when it comes to those with mental health concerns. There are days when we can start waking them up at six o'clock and the getting-dressed process can still be ongoing hours later."

He painted a colourful picture of flying shirts and sweaters. "Usually they belong to ladies who can change their minds like teenagers on a first date. And if they don't like the look of what's in their own wardrobes, they're quite likely to walk into another room in search of something they like better. It's not just the women, though. Norman once went into Annie Lacey-Hallbright's room after she'd gone to breakfast and took a pair of black socks off her bed. I think he must have done it before, because the moment she discovered they were missing, she hurried back to the lounge and confronted him. Not that she got anywhere. Norman pointed out that there were a lot of people wearing black socks that morning, including the matron. Annie went away shaking her head, though I did see her look down at Matron's feet (there were no black socks, of course) when the latter came into the lounge to say, 'Good morning!'

"Annie," continued Alphonso, "is never a problem. She's not one of those who always seem to be in two minds when it comes to what they're going to wear. It's not that she's old-fashioned or anything. In fact, I would describe her as a thoroughly modern ninety-something year-old. Her clothes – sometimes trousers and sometimes a dark, smart skirt – are different every day. The only thing that stays the same is a pearl necklace left to her by her mother."

When I interrupted to suggest that Betsy, of dancing fame, seemed to have something strikingly eye-catching around her neck every day of the week, he gave a cheerful chuckle. "She'd be in for breakfast at the same time as Annie if it weren't for her jewellery.

"Usually, she starts off with some emerald and golden beads she bought in a Delhi bazaar goodness knows how many years ago. Then she puts them back and tries the silver bangles she and Henry collected for their award-winning waltz on one of their more recent trips to Singapore. And if neither of those suits her mood, she'll start dipping into a pile of costume jewellery she picked up at market stalls around the world. You should see it sometime; a sackful of the stuff and it's all as sparkling as the lady herself. Quite frankly I'm never surprised that she has such a hard time making her decisions.

"Sometimes, she'll ask me what I think. She just needs a bit of convincing that she's making a good choice. To be honest, what she's wearing provides a huge source of conversation at Farrow Hall. Hardly a day goes by when someone isn't asking about the background to whatever's hanging around her neck. It does her good to reminisce about her round-the-world travels and the others love to listen to her tales. Like a lot of them, she has a wonderful memory when it comes to the good old days."

Nakita, he said, was another who could dress herself without any kind of fuss; to do anything else would not be in her nature. She had a number of outfits which, as I had noticed, looked very much the same. Neat, schoolmarmish-type kilt or skirt, coupled with a medium grey or light grey cardigan and some frighteningly functional black shoes: lace-ups with leather heels.

"And then there's her handbag," continued Alphonso. "Rather like Mrs Thatcher, she uses it as a prop. In fact, it's verging on an offensive weapon. She clouted me with it the other day when I said that someone other than her should be allowed to choose what they watched on TV that evening. I think it was last Thursday that I decided to give John Huntley a chance to say what he wanted. He never asks for anything, but after I'd heard his son telling him about some upcoming documentary on ancient burial grounds, I felt I should do something about it. I found the right channel at the right time, only Nakita and the other ladies ganged up on the poor man and, of course, on me. They said John would need to wait until he was on his own if he wanted to waste time on that kind of rubbish. They wanted to watch Grace Kelly in *High Society* and, as you've guessed, they had their way. John gave me a look. He didn't want to take that lot on and, quite frankly, neither did I."

His mention of John Huntley prompted me to ask about the men's attire. How come they didn't do as the women in sticking with something more formal than casual?

Alphonso was called to his phone at that point, so I was left to ponder on the matter for myself.

While James Frobisher, who had been born and brought up in Glasgow, always favoured a suit and carried his copy of the Glasgow *Herald* around the place, Norman was one of two or three who stuck with tracksuit bottoms. Norman had plenty of clothes which would not have looked out of place alongside James Frobisher's suit, but his more respectable trousers required braces and he couldn't be bothered with them. And neither could the staff. They gave up on the day he threatened a terrified part-time care worker called Josie with some ancient saying about 'having her guts for garters'.

The Colonel dressed precisely how he might have dressed at his all-male golf club. Old blazer with neatly arranged pocket handkerchief, white shirt, dark grey slacks and socks which bore his initials AJE (Adam Johnson-Edwards). He once told me that his sister, Mildred, gave him a couple of pairs every year and that they came from Savile Row.

I hoped that Norman would know not to take them after the telling-off he had had from Annie Lacey-Hallbright about her missing black socks.

As far as I knew, he had not taken them but, some three weeks after that conversation with Alphonso, the

Colonel stood up in the lounge in front of Alphonso and the majority of the residents to deliver the news that his monogrammed socks were missing.

I was pretty certain that Norman was not guilty of that particular theft, at least not that day. And the reason I knew was because John Huntley had come up to me the moment I arrived to say that the pink socks on Norman's feet belonged to him. And when I apologised on Norman's behalf, John told me that I was not to worry about it. "The last thing I want is to have them back," he said. "My niece sent them over from Canada. The stupid girl must have known that I've never worn pink socks in my life and I have no intention of wearing them while I'm here. My wife must have packed them."

Norman had never been a man for pink socks either. I was surprised that he would have changed his mind and all the more surprised when I learned from Alphonso that he had in fact been guilty of raiding the Colonel's room that very morning and that the monogrammed socks had been his first choice. The crime had not gone undetected for long.

"When I noticed the AJE initials, I told him what he had done and said that he'd better take them off," said Alphonso.

"He wasn't going to take any notice of me but, when I pointed to the initials, he yanked them off at once. He said he certainly didn't put them on deliberately because no one in his family would have dreamed of wearing monogramed socks."

That rang a bell. Years before, Norman had told me how his mother would conveniently dismiss anything she could not afford as "vulgar in the extreme".

Chapter 17: The Other Half

It was not uncommon for a new resident to show signs of improvement at the same time as his/her partner appeared to be struggling.

Dorothy and Bernhard were just one couple who conformed to this pattern, the two having been dependent on each other through sixty years of married life. When Dorothy was admitted to Farrow Hall, there is no question that she benefited from the well-organised routine at the establishment. Equally obvious was the fact that Bernhard was struggling: his life was becoming tougher rather than the reverse.

He admitted as much on a day when he and May Simpson, the golfing lady, were reliving past experiences. They had been joined by Norman who was no different from May in having steered well clear of the afternoon yoga class. I, meantime, was sitting on the periphery of that group as I scanned a list of songs I had been asked to play during Millicent Smith's ninety-ninth birthday tea. Since there were at least three songs that I had not played in months, I was busy running through them in my head and, because of it, I did no more than lend half an ear to the conversation.

Bernhard had plenty to say about his experiences.

"We were muddling along all right at home, only it was not really all right," he began.

May intervened to say that "muddling along" was the perfect description of how things had been for her after her husband had gone into Squire Place, the home where he had died in 2009. "So how are you managing to make things work, Bernhard?" she asked.

"Things have been pretty disastrous for about seven years, now," he sighed. "While Dorothy was living at home, I managed to steer her in the right direction and, as I say, we muddled along fine – at least until the day she left the cooking to me and disappeared without my noticing it. That was a disaster of a night if ever there was one. She went out of our flat and, though everyone else in the block had been primed to watch out for her, someone had let her out of the main entrance. I managed to catch up with her when she was about a hundred yards down the road, only then I had the devil of a job persuading her to come home.

"When we finally got back to the flat, I smelt burning. Straightaway, I knew it was the lamb chops I'd been cooking and, funnily enough, the smell of burning was enough to bring Dorothy to her senses. The chops were ruined but one of my neighbours had rung my daughter, Jessie, to say there was a fire in our kitchen. and Dorothy and I had disappeared. I could have done without that.

"Anyhow, Jessie came round about five minutes later and she was exasperated to say the least. I told her that it was all my fault, but what I didn't tell her was how much worse her mother had become in the space of no more than a couple of weeks. Jessie knew, though. She'd been telling me for ages that Dorothy needed to go into a home.

"We got away with more of that muddling along until Dorothy disappeared again. This time, it was a man delivering parcels who had let her out and the police who found her in the middle of the road. They brought her back and said that she was lucky to be alive. The way they said it made me feel guilty."

When Bernhard felt obliged to ring his children with the latest news before they rang him, they took charge.

"They just took over at that point. They booked her into Farrow Hall and that was that."

"And is it making things any easier?" persisted May.

Bernhard seemed to sense what she was thinking. "You mean for me rather than for Dorothy?"

"Yes, Bernhard," she said. "I'm wondering how it's working for you. I'm only asking because I've noticed that you've lost a bit of weight. You need to look after yourself, you know. I lost weight when Phillip went into his home. I could cook all right, but I couldn't be bothered with it. For a while, I was going to see him every afternoon and, by the time I got back, I didn't have the energy for too much else. It was one of my sons who told me I needed to get a grip of myself. He started organising packs of ready-meals for me from some local farm shop and I stuck with them, at least until I came in here. Actually, that reminds me. I hope someone cancelled them."

At this point, May seemed to realise, with a start, that she had created an unnecessary diversion when Bernhard had been in full swing with his story.

"Why on earth didn't you stop me?" she said to him. "Here I am going on about me when you were about to say how you've been finding things since you've been on your own."

"Don't you worry, May," he said. "It's been interesting for me to hear what you've been saying. It tells me that I need to get myself organised. In fact, I think I could do with a few of those ready-meals. I'll ask Jessie about them.

"But to answer your question, I found it quite relaxing at the start, coming in here, I mean, and having tea and cake and chatting with Dorothy and all the other residents and their visitors. That side of things has always been fine. It's just the leaving bit where it all goes wrong. You've probably seen what Dorothy's like when I have to go. Not always but quite a lot of the time."

I chipped in at this point to offer a bit of sympathy; I had seen Bernhard age by the minute on those days when he tried to take his leave of a ballistic Dorothy. "There's no question that you have a harder time than most. I always admire your patience when it comes to explaining why you have to go. It can't be easy."

Our conversation suddenly came to a halt.

Norman was awake, the yoga class was over, Dorothy was making her way across the room and

Mabel's birthday cake, the centre-piece of the tea trolley arrangement, was being wheeled into the room. It was time for me to get back to my post.

Mabel, who looked younger than her ninety-nine years at that point, stood up and said that everyone was welcome to a slice of her chocolate cake. She handed it round and described with pride how her daughter, Emily, had taken the recipe from a book which had been in the family since 1856. "My mother would bake the cake for my sisters and me when we were little and I used to bake it for my daughters. Now Emily is baking that same recipe for her children – as well as for me, of course. Long may the tradition last!"

Residents and visitors gave her a round of applause before starting to debate the respective merits or demerits of their own cake-baking. Mabel's son, Larry, offered everyone a glass of wine and a merry afternoon was had by all until the time came for Bernhard to go home. Dorothy, on what had up until then been a delightful afternoon, was not at her best. She said it was ridiculous that she couldn't go back to her own flat and eventually made such an extraordinary rumpus that Alphonso had to intervene. Alphonso asked her to write out the following day's lunch menu on the grounds that her handwriting was so much better than anyone else's and Bernhard made his escape. He was sweating.

The following day there was a particularly sad exchange between the two of them.

"I've got to go now, Dorothy," he said at four o'clock.

"I think I'll come with you."

"We know that's not possible, Dorothy. I can't look after you."

"I can look after myself,"

"No, you can't."

"We can look after each other," she persisted.

"No," returned Bernhard. "We're too old to look after each other."

"Nonsense," she declared.

At that moment, Dorothy was distracted by a resident's wife who was trying to help her husband switch from his wheelchair to a regular chair.

"Who's that lady?" asked Dorothy,

"It's that gentleman's wife," replied Bernhard.

"Don't be silly," she answered in somewhat imperious tones. "Why would she be married to him? He's no use to her. He can barely move."

Bernhard, by this time, was dying a thousand deaths as her voice rang out round the room.

He left as Dorothy continued to rage. He could take no more.

The nursing staff would often tell him that he did not need to appear on a daily basis, especially with winter approaching, but he could not stop himself. He had tried staying away but the guilt factor was too much. In his culture – Bernhard was born and brought up in Austria – it was bad enough to have put someone in a home, let alone stop visiting him or her.

Winter was creeping up on Farrow Hall quicker than ever that year and, with the first snowfall, I went to see if the window at the end of one of the corridors – it was Professor Perkins's end, and a few enquiries had revealed that she was asleep – permitted a view of the snow settling on the hills. Since it was an even better view than I had anticipated, I returned to the lounge and suggested that some of the ladies might want to go along and see it for themselves.

While I stayed at the piano, knocking out "Let it snow, Let it Snow, Let it Snow" (a song apparently written at the height of a Californian summer) the advance party set out. It consisted of Nakita and Alicia, along with a gentleman who had never previously evinced an interest in joining in with anything.

Annie Lacey-Hallbright, Betsy and Dorothy followed on ten minutes later, with the delay down to Betsy's concerns as to whether or not she should take her handbag and, if so, which handbag it should be.

The second party were back in their seats and chattering excitedly about the delights of the snow-spattered hills when I started to wonder about the whereabouts of the first group. "They must have taken a different route," said Dorothy. Since any different route would have included a trip through the garden via an emergency exit, I disappeared in a hurry to ask Professor Perkins if she had seen them at all.

Professor Perkins was awake at this point and working on the roof of Jenners in her Edinburgh jigsaw. She was dealing with the very top floor of that once-famous department store which, by now, could be well on its way to becoming a boutique hotel. When I asked if she had seen the residents in question, she could not have been more agitated by the interruption. "I saw Dorothy, Annie and Betsy, if that's what those women are called, but no one else came my way, thank heavens. In fact, I would thank you not to send anyone else down my corridor because the reason I sit here, in case no one has ever made you aware of it, is to get a bit of peace. Please advise everyone else that the snow has melted."

Though the snow was coming down more heavily than ever, I made an appropriate apology and she returned to work.

Matron was rather more helpful. I left the whereabouts of the missing residents to her and, in no time at all, she put her head round the lounge door with the answer. All members of the advance party had apparently ended up in their rooms, having clean forgotten where they were going and why.

Once they had reassembled in the lounge, Dorothy felt duty-bound to regale them with details of what they had missed. Two of them were grateful, Nakita was not. She was infuriated by Dorothy's happy feedback and, as a result, was looking for trouble.

After making a meal of studying her watch, she interrupted Dorothy with some news. "It's ten past two and there's no sign of Bernhard. Shouldn't he be here by now?"

"What time do you think it is?" said Dorothy. "The clock on the wall says it's only five past."

"But he's usually bang on two, isn't he?"

"Is he? Oh yes, I'm sure you're right, I hope nothing's happened to him. What do you think, Nakita?

"I don't know. It's just that it struck me that he was late. I mean, it's well after five past now."

Dorothy leapt from her chair.

"I'll go and see if he's in the hall."

When she returned alone, Nakita told her to go back and look again. There were a couple more abortive searches, at the end of which Matron involved herself in the conversation and said it was far too soon to be worried. The traffic was bad and she was sure Bernhard would be with her before too long.

Which he was. At twenty past two, to be precise. He limped in and whatever was left of Dorothy's frenzy evaporated.

The couple sat down near the piano and, straightaway, Dorothy told Bernhard about the snow.

It triggered a host of "Do you remember" stories from both of them, with Matron sitting down to join in with a reminiscence of her own. She had been working in the A & E department at Edinburgh's old Royal

Infirmary at the time and had taken advantage of a brief break to walk across the Meadows on what was a sunny, snowy day. On the way back, she slipped on the pavement and broke her wrist – just in time for the start of her next shift. The doctor in A & E, a rather surly piece of work, had taken one look and said, "We've got enough to do without this."

Matron's story ended just seconds before she was called to attend a room-bound patient. She darted up from her chair but, before she went, she suggested that Bernhard should be on his way home. The weather was getting worse.

Possibly for the first time, Dorothy did not make any kind of fuss. "Yes, Bernhard," she said, "Matron's right. We've had a lovely afternoon, so off you go. Enjoy your supper and I'll see you tomorrow."

Bernhard agreed that they had had the best of days and, after giving her a little hug, he was on his way. For the first time in months, he was smiling as he exited the room. He whispered a conspiratorial, "That was a nice change," as he shuffled past the piano.

They never did see each other again. Apparently, he had a stroke in Tesco on his way home later that evening and collapsed by the tills. The manager called for help and, in less than half an hour, Bernhard was in hospital. At A & E, they did what they could for him, but more strokes followed and he died two days later.

For weeks afterwards, Dorothy talked of how he would be joining them for tea. Yet well though the staff handled the situation – they were always good in such circumstances – no one did more to turn sobs into smiles than Nakita. Every afternoon, she danced kindly attention on her friend, scurrying to and fro with cups of tea made by her good self (as opposed to her nastier self).

Chapter 18: A Bridge Too Far

The tunes on this July evening started with 'Music of the Night' from *The Phantom of the Opera*. Not my version but a rendition by a well-known cellist, Josif Moran, who, to all-round disbelief, had agreed to come to Farrow Hall. There is no question that music of all kinds can affect a dementia victim as much if not more than anything else and, as Moran's music filled the air, it was as if the strings' vibrations were re-setting lost minds.

Donald McIntyre, a charmer of a gentleman who was well-known for guffawing his way around Farrow Hall, was transformed. All of a sudden, he was at peace with the world and doing a bit of gentle conducting with the spoon he had taken from his pocket. I saw Matron elbowing Alphonso by way of drawing his attention to the resident's reactions.

This concert had come about when the cellist was staying in Fife where he was enjoying a golfing holiday before performing at Edinburgh's Usher Hall.

I had met him at a hotel reception desk in Sweden several months before when we found ourselves waiting in vain for a receptionist who never came. We started to discuss the travelling involved in our respective jobs, mine as a sports writer and his as a musician and, after standing around for an unconscionably long time, we adjourned to an adjoining coffee shop. (We put our luggage, though not the cello, behind the desk and left a note to advise whoever it was that was meant to be signing in the new arrivals where he or she would find her latest guests.) While in the restaurant, we came to the following arrangement: Josif would sort out a couple of tickets for a colleague and myself for the recital he was giving two days later in a church hall before playing at the Concert Hall in Stockholm. I, in turn, would give him a couple of Court One tickets for Wimbledon where I used to work on a daily diary for my newspaper.

When the church concert never happened because of repairs to the masonry – some stones from the spire had landed alarmingly close to the entrance – he gave me a ring and said he would try to get me tickets for the Concert Hall in the city instead. And when he rang back to say that every ticket was taken, he asked if there was anything else he could do for me instead.

More by way of a joke than anything else, I suggested that he might like to play a few short pieces at Farrow Hall on his forthcoming trip to Scotland. I explained a bit about Farrow Hall and how it would provide an amazing interlude in the residents' lives,

He smiled broadly and, far from trying to wriggle his way out of this improbable invitation, he said, "I'd love to!"

"Are you sure you'd love to?"

"Yes, sure. I'm playing a new composition at the Usher Hall and I need to give it a try in front of a live audience. As yet, nothing's been arranged, so a trip to Farrow Hall would save my team having to sort something out."

It was all faintly ridiculous, but Matron and Alphonso seized on the idea, as did Mr Marquis, who felt that such a visit could only add to his home's prestige. He was somewhat alarmed that it was a bit of a last-minute affair – this was 4 June and the concert was set for 2 July – but he got cracking just the same.

First, he compiled his invitation list.

Since Farrow Hall could accommodate twenty outsiders in addition to the forty-seven residents and their visitors, he decided that Edinburgh's Lord Provost, in all his regalia, would add a bit of clout, as would the vicar. Going on from there, he decided on a handful of local councillors, a couple of elders from the church round the corner, and five committee members, all of them women, from the Literary Society. (Presumably he was viewing them as potential residents.)

The invitations complete, he oversaw the maintenance men as they set up a stage at the end of the dining room before oiling a stubborn set of sliding doors between the dining area and the lounge. At the same time, the boss and his son cleared out the library so that Moran and his fellow musicians, along with everyone else, could have pre-concert drinks.

Jenni, the oldest grandchild, was asked to design and print a programme, while her three siblings were charged with making people welcome and passing round drinks.

The excitement spread throughout the home and, yes, it turned out that Nakita had not only played the cello in her schooldays but been a mainstay of the school orchestra. Only Dorothy was kind enough to ask for further details, though so loudly did Nakita proceed to dispense them that others could not fail to hear. She had kept on playing until she and her husband, Eric, had the third of their three children and moved to a bigger house. At that point, she asked Eric to store the cello somewhere safe while the children were young and he selected a dry and airy cellar. What he failed to consider was that it was already serving as home to a family of mice. They chewed a hole in the case before starting on the instrument itself. "So that was the end of my cello," she said. "A pity, because I played it well."

Someone mumbled "How predictable!" and, at a guess, I would have said that it was one or other of Alicia Hemple or Annie Lacey-Hallbright, both of whom were close at hand.

The big night arrived. For those residents who were not sufficiently mobile to join the drinks party, the arrival of the various dignitaries was an event in itself. They came in their finest outfits, with the five ladies from the Literary Society having no doubt come to some agreement about giving outings to long-forgotten hats.

One was a purple creation, two were pink, a fourth was more turban than hat – a pale green concoction – while the fifth was a simple beret decorated with a miniature spray of fresh flowers. Its owner said that the flowers had been plucked from her garden.

Meanwhile, there were three men in kilts, one of whom was identified by Nakita (wrongly, as it turned out) as a male councillor said to have had his kilt let out at the waist at the taxpayer's expense. Josif, the star of the evening, was in evening dress, with his fellow musicians more casually attired.

Ten minutes ahead of the concert's seven o'clock start, Jenni handed round the programmes as the other children shepherded the guests through to the smartly-labelled seats.

Mr Marquis leapt onto the stage at the appointed hour and explained how proud he was to be able to welcome such a fine musician to Farrow Hall. He then reeled off the names of some of the great concert halls where Josif Moran had played. "There's the Carnegie Hall, the Royal Bernhard Hall, the Royal Opera House in Sydney, and the Stockholm Concert Hall," he began, before delivering a line which had the visiting musician chortling delightedly. "And as from tonight, he, Josif Moran, will be able to add Farrow Hall to that list!

"Now, can I please ask you to welcome our great cellist to the stage."

Where Mr Marquis had enjoyed leaping on to the podium, Josif arrived at the stage's foot and came to an abrupt halt. He beamed from ear to ear as he addressed his audience. "Can anyone lend me a walking-stick?"

Walking-sticks shot up all over the room as he explained, amidst laughter, how he had hurt his knee climbing the seven hills of Edinburgh. In the event, no walking-sticks were required. Nakita had stolen a march on the walking-stick brigade by whipping the footstool from under May Simpson's leg and introducing it as a bottom step. Problem solved, if only on a temporary basis.

Josif nodded in Nakita's direction before thanking Mr Marquis for his opening address and explained how he would begin with 'Music of the Night' from *The Phantom of the Opera*. He planned to follow up with a couple of other popular melodies before giving an airing to a new piece, the one he had composed himself but which he had never performed in public before. He had yet to lay bow on string but already his audience was hooked.

He followed 'Music of the Night' with 'Amazing Grace', before allowing a mini-interval in which the audience could react. Everyone clapped with a youthful enthusiasm, almost until they could clap no more. Yet there came a moment, five minutes into 'There's a Place for Us' from *West Side Story,* when they were called upon to be altogether more energetic.

In the middle of a particularly powerful passage, the cello's bridge parted company from the main body of the instrument and sprang into the body of the lounge.

The shocked silence was broken by an angry Professor Perkins, the lady who had been similarly out of order at our Christmas Concert. She contributed a raucous, "Get on with it!"

Josif looked at her, helplessly, as the more able-bodied members of the audience got down on their hands and knees in a major search operation. My son, Logan, who was up from London and had been regaling Norman with updates on golf and rugby, joined in. After an inordinate amount of noisy scuffling, which involved Nakita telling the ladies from the Literary Society, "You're only getting in the way", the purplehatted member of their quintette held the bridge up as high as she could for Nakita and everyone else to see. It had come to rest in her open handbag.

While cello and bridge were being reunited backstage, Mr Marquis delivered glasses of water or wine to the performers. The twins did the same for the audience and May had words with Nakita in connection with the pilfering of her footstool. "Don't you dare do that to me again!" she said. Nakita would have remonstrated with her, only there were calls for silence as Mr Moran took delivery of his cello and sat down.

The concert resumed without further ado, with the piece which our cellist had composed himself, 'The Still of Winter', raising goose-pimples all round.

The evening had been a resounding success in everyone's eyes, save for Josif's. When the cheers came, he responded with a series of bows, each of which came across as more of an apology than anything else.

I caught up with him on his way into the library for the parting drinks and snacks which Mr Marquis had arranged for the musicians and the visiting local luminaries. Josif winced as he thanked me. "For a bridge to take flight in mid-concert like that is one of the most embarrassing things that can happen, I'm afraid. I'm so very sorry."

I said there was no need to apologise. The evening had exceeded my wildest dreams and what had happened couldn't have happened in a better place. The residents had loved their involvement and, as for the lady in the purple hat, she was probably heading for home with a story she could tell for the rest of her days.

He managed a smile. "Maybe I'll manage to see it like that one day, only this isn't that day."

I rather hoped that his Wimbledon experience – it was going to be his first – would hasten the process.

In the world of tennis, snapping strings and racket frames were all part of the game.

Chapter 19: The Last Laugh

Angus, the table tennis coach who visited Farrow Hall every second week with his son Jim, needed an extra pair of hands with his Wednesday morning class. He asked if I would take a turn in hitting with a couple of the residents but, more than that, he wanted me to watch Nancy. This, incidentally, had nothing to do with Nancy's age, for she was only in her seventies at a time when there was a story on YouTube about an Australian lady by the name of Dorothy who was competing in a world Over-80s table-tennis tournament when she was a hundred.

The reason Nancy was so special was allied to her dementia. Though she could not string a sentence together, she could sustain a rally of thirty, forty or even fifty shots while all the time roaring with laughter.

Angus, whose mother had stayed at Farrow Hall not too long before, had offered the fortnightly table tennis class by way of giving something back to a home where his mother had spent a happy last few months. His suspicion that such a class might work had nothing to do with his late mother, who left sporting activities to the male side of the family. Rather was it the sight of the Yoga teacher struggling through the door one day with a bag of plastic rackets and sponge balls. He plied the teacher with questions and, as he had half-expected, she said that residents who had grown up hitting a ball of one kind or another were quick to rediscover that dormant talent. She also captured his interest with news of how research in Japan has provided clinical evidence that table tennis can affect five different portions of the brain simultaneously, thereby promoting "a sense of awakening" among Alzheimer's and dementia victims.

Angus's and Jim's first action on arriving at Farrow Hall that Wednesday was to rearrange the breakfast tables. They pushed them together in sets of two before adding one of those stretch-to-fit-any-size-of-table nets, an invention with the potential to play havoc with traditional dining in everything from royal households to the most humble of homes. Usually, the classes started at nine thirty but today, because the hairdresser was doing her rounds, it was ten thirty.

Barely had father and son finished setting things up than the residents filed in, with Angus handing out bats at the door. Four ladies and two gentlemen – they included Norman, who promptly stored his bat behind a large clock on the mantlepiece – were in the mood to play; two other ladies and another couple of gentlemen just fancied being in a room where something was going on; while there was a fifth gentleman for whom the sound of bat on ball did the same for him as music might do for another.

"Will Nakita and Dorothy come along?" I asked.

"No chance," said a bemused Angus. "I think that Dorothy could have been persuaded to come if she had wandered in on her own, but Nakita announced that table tennis was not 'their thing' and added that all of the recruits were wasting their time – and mine. She then gave me chapter and verse on how good she would have been if she had taken it up."

"That's Nakita all right," I said.

Nancy apart, the other more active members of the class were Alicia, along with Moira Jones and Daisy Edgerton from upstairs, and Samuel, a retired GP.

Sam, the doctor, was soon into his stride, enjoying the beginnings of one good rally after another in the company of Jim. The only trouble was that he would catch the ball after six or seven shots and explain that he needed to stop. In his eyes at least, the handful of spectators who were sitting with their backs to the wall were his patients and he thought they would take a dim view of how he was keeping them waiting.

Among the women, Alicia was a natural but needed a quick-witted care worker to catch her on those occasions when she dived for a ball which she would have struggled to reach twenty years before. Moira Jones had been a useful tennis player in her day and was in the same league as Alicia in terms of talent while being woefully short of concentration. As for Daisy, she was stymied in her efforts to play well because she had a poor-quality playing companion – me. Norman suddenly took an interest, saying that Daisy was clearly a member of the first team and that I was holding her back.

Daisy agreed. With a shrug of the shoulders, she drew Norman's attention to how I had suddenly disappeared under the table, and never mind that I was merely collecting a couple of balls which had wedged themselves between the wall and the leg of a serving trolley. When I reappeared, Daisy was prepared to give me "one last chance".

If there was one area where every resident – player or non-player – excelled, it applied to fielding the runaway, bouncing balls. Without exception, they made it their business to try and catch them before returning them to the nearest player. This even applied to those in wheelchairs who would bend down almost further than was safely possible. Angus said that it mirrored the situation in the primary schools where he taught; picking up the balls seemed to be as much a part of the fun as any other aspect of the experience.

With Daisy declaring that I had wasted my last chance, I left her chatting to Norman on the subject of where she had learnt her forehand as I sat down to watch Angus's star pupil.

Nancy was a stocky, upright lady, her face crisscrossed with laughter lines. Just as Betsy always dressed as if she were ready to get up and dance, so Nancy was kitted out for sport. On this occasion, she was wearing a navy sweater and navy slacks along with a pair of matching trainers. As for her silvery hair, that was tied back with a white headband.

I marvelled at the rallies she was having with Angus. It seemed that she never missed, with one well-placed shot coming hard on the heels of another. Rallies of thirty shots made her laugh, but never as much as the ones when Angus would announce that they had passed the fifty mark.

About twenty minutes into the session, when they were in the throes of a rally to end all rallies, a couple of care workers took over from Angus with the counting.

"Sixty-four, sixty-five, sixty-six, sixty-seven," they chanted, before moving on to the first half of the 'sixty-eight'. Alas, they got no further than that first syllable thanks to the visitor who chose that very moment to make an ostentatious entry. He had recognised Angus and, much to Angus's irritation, he had assumed that he would want to stop everything to chat to him.

His opening gambit, after he had looked at Nancy and the other table tennis players, was wholly inappropriate and accompanied by a sneer.

"So, Angus, you're getting in some practice for this evening's league match, are you?"

Angus took a deep breath as if about to give the fellow the kind of response he deserved. Then he plonked his bat on the table and smiled.

"Just my luck," he said. "Have I drawn you in the first round?"

"Yes, it's just come up on my mobile."

"OK," said Angus, "but what are you doing here?"

"It's my father; he's recovering from a hip operation and my sister decided that he needed to stay at Farrow Hall for a few days before going home. Damned nuisance as far as I'm concerned but I suppose it can't be helped."

Though it would have been nice had he spared a thought for his father as well as himself, no one said as much. As the interloper left, Angus merely raised his eyebrows and apologised for the chap's poor manners.

"Sorry about that," he began. "First, he ruined that rally we were all enjoying, and then he gives me the bad news that I've drawn him in the first round of the league. He's the best player in the club and in all the years I've played him, I've never won. He's a wily old so-and-so!"

No sooner had Angus and Nancy returned to the business of the day than there was a second diversion, one so alarming as to put people in mind of stags and crashing antlers in a David Attenborough documentary.

The sound effects were down to a couple of residents using their zimmers as weapons. Old Bertie McFie, the one who liked the sound of bats on balls, had been leaving the room when Lady Jane Smith, who had been keeping an eye on everything, battered a nearby zimmer into his. Not once but three times. As far as she was concerned, the zimmer which Bertie was gripping belonged to her. Angus stepped in when Bertie was on the point of giving her Ladyship a kick and Norman said that he was going to call the police. An uneasy peace ensued which lasted all of five minutes before Interruption Number Three.

This one was down to Nakita. As she appeared in the doorway, arms akimbo, she announced that the table tennis should have stopped half an hour before and that Angus and Jim would need to put the tables back in their rightful places at once. She and Dorothy had been charged with laying out the napkins for lunch and they would need to get started.

Nancy stopped laughing and gave Nakita a glare. "Go away!" she instructed.

Though Nancy's sentence was on the short side, it nonetheless conveyed everything she wanted to say to her annoying fellow-resident.

Angus was so impressed with Nancy's speech that he weighed in himself, advising Nakita that there would be one last rally on each of the tables.

Each of the rallies was too long as far as Nakita was concerned and, as they finally came to a full-stop, so she hurried round confiscating the balls. That done, she hid them in a teapot on the granite work surface which had been cleaned by Belinda before breakfast, while Angus and Jim were busy telling Nancy and the others that they would make it up to them the next time.

That at least twelve balls had finished up in Nakita's teapot was something I forgot to mention until Angus appeared in the lounge the following day. He didn't have to spell out why he was back.

"I'm so sorry," I said. "Nakita put all the table tennis balls into a teapot on the sideboard . . . I'll go and get them."

As I decanted them into his sports-bag, I remembered to ask how he had fared in his league game.

"I won," he said, "and I can honestly say that it was all down to Nancy."

"Down to Nancy?"

"Well, it was something I was about to explain to you yesterday when you were having trouble hitting with Daisy. The trouble was that there were so many interruptions that I never got round to it.

"What I wanted to tell you is that there's an art in playing with the residents. It's up to you to place the ball in the optimum position for them to be able to hit it back. A touch of top-spin is what's needed. You have to be endlessly precise – and so far was I into that accurate-hitting mode that I was able to carry on where I left off when I came up against Alex."

Having digested the above, I asked Angus if Alex had apologised to him for the way he had sneered at his practice session.

"That was never going to happen," he chuckled. "Nor, for that matter, am I expecting Nakita to say sorry for her remark about my table tennis sessions being an all-round waste of time. Personally, I've never stopped learning since they began."

Chapter 20: A Taste of Trouble

Hamish McMillan, who lived no more than five houses up the road from Farrow Hall and had his name on the honours board at the local tennis club more times than anyone else, was a hale and hearty 85-year-old until the day he went up a ladder – his neighbours said that the ladder was as old as he was – to replace a light bulb. In his haste to test the light, he fell on the way down and broke a leg. Norman, as you might expect, told him he would be back in the tennis club's first team before he knew it.

Hamish seemed to be thinking along the same lines. To him, the accident was nowhere near as big a deal as his neighbours were making out. When, on the day of his arrival, I heard Alphonso asking about the fall, he brought the subject to a speedy conclusion by saying, "I think I'm to be congratulated on getting the bulb changed."

Leg apart, Hamish was looking much better than when I saw him in the village coffee shop following the death of his wife, Peggy, some months before. (She had contracted pneumonia after a hip procedure went awry.)

I happened to be having a coffee with a fellow walker on the day Hamish returned after that sad happening. He was just putting his head around the coffee shop's door when he seemed to be having second thoughts. Then, though, he was swept in automatically by a party of chattering church gardeners.

They made way for him to go up to the counter before them and, as he was waiting to give his order, so a retired lawyer who was on his way out said a perfunctory, "I was sorry to hear about Peggy." At that, Sue, who ran the coffee shop with her mother, Kathy, cut short the business of sprinkling chocolate over someone's cappuccino to turn the lawyer's remark into something more adequate. "I think we were all very sorry to hear about Peggy," she said. Her comment prompted multiple cries of 'Hear, hear!' from pensioners, students and young mums alike – and that was the moment Hamish's face started to light up. He recognised that he was among friends and, as he came and sat next to me, I recognised the extraordinary role that can be played in a community by a good coffee shop.

Hamish returned regularly to the coffee shop after that and, in what was a delightful coincidence, he and a couple of his coffee-shop acquaintances were now overlapping at Farrow Hall. John Huntley had fallen off a garden wall, while Colonel Johnson-Edwards had been knocked over by a dog. (Since the Colonel was no longer wearing a boot on his broken foot, it struck me that he would probably have been back at his home but for his crush on May Simpson.)

The three men were enjoying a reunion in the Farrow Hall lounge when they were interrupted by young Tommy McMillan, Hamish's seven-year-old grandson who, along with assorted siblings, lived in the house next door but one to his. Tommy looked pleased with himself as he produced a grand box of chocolates from a John Lewis carrier-bag.

"This is for you, Grandpa," he said, as he put it on the table between the trio and the piano.

"Are you sure it's for me?"

"Yes," said Tommy. "Mum said I could bring it down here once she'd wrapped it up, but then she went to work without wrapping it up and Dad said I could bring it down here anyway. I think I was getting in his way."

Hamish, an old school gentleman if ever there were one, patted the child on the head before taking hold of the box and removing its outer layer of cellophane. He opened the lid before passing it back to Tommy. "I think you should offer these round to everyone else in the room first," he said. "Perhaps you should start with the residents at the back."

I half wondered if Hamish was merely doing what his son-in-law had done in hitting on something to keep the child occupied while he was busy with something else.

It was impossible to tell whether or not John Huntley was happy with the idea of not having immediate access to the chocolates, but I did notice that the Colonel was not best pleased. He had bent forward to study what was on offer on the purple lid and, judging from his sudden smile, it struck me that he had come face to face with an old favourite. Nor was I the only person watching him. May Simpson, I thought, was eyeing him somewhat critically.

Once Tommy had embarked on his round-the-room delivery, Hamish made light-hearted mention of how his daughter seemed to have forgotten that her father didn't really like chocolates, especially the Cadbury's Milk Tray variety. Mr Huntley said that whether you liked it or not, chocolates were what you tended to get when you broke something; he had been given a tin of them after his fall. The Colonel, on the other hand, said that his family had produced a potted plant which was the last thing he needed.

Professor Perkins, who had been wheeled into the room to look for her copy of *The Times*, promptly and proudly let everyone know that she was actually older than Milk Tray. "I was born in 1910 and they came out in 1915," she said.

That was not the end of her contribution to the chocolate debate. She called Tommy across so that she could look in the box and see if she recognised any of the contents from her childhood. She peered through her monocle. "Where is the Coffee Cream, I wonder? There's no sign of it on the lid and I can't see one inside."

Guy Clutterbuck was able to inform her that the coffee chocolates, like the Turkish Delight, an old favourite of his, were probably a thing of the past.

"I wonder if they ask for people's opinions when they do something like that?" said Professor Perkins.

"Well, they certainly didn't want mine," said Guy. "I got my wife to write in and complain and we got a note back saying that it was to do with the manufacturing process having moved from England to Poland or something."

Since the piano was no longer getting my full attention, and since the last thing I wanted was for Young Tommy to think that I was too busy to qualify for a chocolate, I closed the piano lid and joined in with what was fast becoming a healthy if rather noisy debate. At one point, when things went quiet, I asked a couple of residents, who looked as if they wanted to venture an opinion, if they had a favourite. James Frobisher, the *Glasgow Herald* reader, said that he liked the old lime edition. Maisie merely pointed at the box without being any more specific. Norman said he liked "the chocolate one" and May Simpson said that she was a fan of the Hazelnut Swirl. The Colonel interjected with the news that he liked that one too. Simultaneously, he nodded his head as if to suggest that this was a classic example of great minds thinking alike. May Simpson looked irritated.

Tommy was continuing to make good progress but, after I had spotted Major Briggs putting one chocolate in his mouth and another under the rim of his saucer, I began to wonder if there would be enough to go round. The concern became altogether more acute when I noticed Tommy surreptitiously stuffing a couple of chocolates – I couldn't see which – into his pocket as he crossed between Major Briggs and Annie Lacey-Hallbright. Annie took a peach chocolate and put it on her table for a moment while she picked up Agatha James's walking stick. In the time it took, Agatha whipped Annie's chocolate from the table and ate it herself. It was typical of Annie that she wasn't about to make a big deal of the situation. She simply looked heavenwards and said, "Blow me!" before helping herself to something else. Maisie took a chocolate without so much as looking at it and Guy declared that chocolates were not very good for any of them before taking two for himself.

At this point, Tommy stopped off next to his grandfather to tell him that there were only five chocolates left and that there were at least four chocolate-less people at the front of the room.

"Well that's all right," said Hamish, "You can forget me."

"And me," said John Huntley.

"Me too," I volunteered.

"And you, Colonel?" queried Hamish.

"Well," said the Colonel, "if there are five chocolates left over for the four residents I can see at the front – Nakita, Dorothy, Alicia and May – it's okay for me to have one."

Hamish looked as if he was struggling to believe what he was hearing but gave him the go-ahead just the same. The Colonel then proceeded to take the very chocolate to which May Simpson had given a mention, the Hazelnut Swirl. I pondered, momentarily, on whether he was forgetful, plain greedy, or both.

Tommy, meantime, had moved on to the left-over residents and, predictably, his dealings with Nakita, the first of them, were not exactly straightforward. "Who took the fudge ones, that's what I'd like to know?" she demanded.

Honest Tommy owned up at once.

"I took them, but it's okay, you can have them back. They're in my pocket."

He took them out of his pocket, along with a rotting apple core, and laid them on the table in front of her.

Nakita started in her seat and looked disgusted. Tommy began to cry.

"It's all right, Tommy," she said. "You just keep those for yourself and I'll choose another." She said she would take the one shaped like a strawberry as soon as she had wiped the boy's hands and eyes with a paper napkin.

Dorothy, who was sitting next to her, said that she had had her eye on the strawberry one. Nakita gave her a glare but Alicia, who was next in line, said that she knew how to sort out what sounded like an unnecessary argument. She said she would eat the strawberry one herself and she did.

Alicia's reaction put Nakita and Dorothy back on the same side. They were as peeved as each other that Alicia should have taken such peremptory action, and crosser than ever when they discovered that the identical chocolates on which they had agreed from the remaining three were playing havoc with their dentures.

Tommy picked up the final chocolate in his supposedly clean fingers and handed it to May, only before he handed it over, he added an impressive bit of history as to why she would not be getting the chocolate of her choice. "I heard you say that you liked the Hazelnut Swirl but I'm afraid the Colonel took the last one."

"I saw that for myself, thank you Tommy."

The Colonel cringed and started to fiddle with his shoelaces.

Seconds earlier, I had noticed Matron standing in the doorway with her hands on her hips.

"Hamish," she called. "Those chocolates weren't for you at all. They were for the staff. Your daughter's just rung to say that you don't like chocolates and that you'd happily hand them over."

Hamish looked anything but concerned at being at the centre of such mischief.

"I'm afraid it's a bit late for that," he said. Yet just as he was about to hand her the empty box, he was struck by its weight.

"Hang on a moment, Matron. I don't think the situation's as bad as you think it is."

He whipped the empty tray from the top to reveal a second layer and, had he been holding on to the wrong end of a red-hot poker, he could not have shoved it into Matron's hands more quickly.

"You're welcome to them," he said. "If the second layer's anything like the first, you can expect nothing but trouble."

Chapter 21: Warning Strokes

The beginning of the end for Norman came in the summer of 2014 after he had fallen and injured a hip. On the doctor's advice, he was dispatched to hospital. But well though the operation went – it did not involve a full-scale hip replacement – the after-treatment was not worthy of the surgeon's labours. The trouble was that there was no such thing as an orthopaedic-cum-dementia ward; you could have an orthopaedic condition or dementia problems, but not both.

They took him to the orthopaedic ward, where Suzi, Patrick and I arrived in time to find our patient waking up and making frantic attempts to pull out every one of the gadgets and tubes the surgeon had so carefully inserted. Straight away, I reported the news to the girl at the nurse's station outside the ward door. (Whoever thought of putting nurses' stations outside a ward rather than inside?)

The nurse slotted everything back in place but when, ten minutes later, Norman returned to the demolition work, I sought more help. By then, a senior male nurse had taken over at the desk. I could see that he was dealing with some administrative work but, to me at least, the situation was urgent. "I'm sorry," I began, "but my husband's at it again: he's pulling out all the tubes and now he's trying to get out of bed."

Ever so slowly, the nurse laid down his pen.

"He's quite a man, your husband," he replied, with an irritating air of nonchalance. That said, he returned to his paperwork.

As luck would have it, the original girl reappeared, only by then Norman was sufficiently awake to be in a foul temper as well. Another patient's visitors, three of whom I vaguely recognised, assailed me with worried looks. I got the impression, maybe wrongly, that they were expecting me to come across and say something. However, since they might not have known about Norman's dementia, the situation was going to take too much explaining and, quite frankly, I was not in the mood.

There were only four beds in that ward and, as we left, I remember one of the patients who had yet to have his operation, calling me aside. He asked a concerned, "Has your husband just been badly affected by his hip procedure?" I assured him that that was not the case and that he himself had nothing to worry about. It was one more happening to suggest that Norman was maybe not where he should have been.

With higher sides having been added to the hospital bed, Norman somehow survived the next couple of days before being taken back to Farrow Hall where the first thing I did was to beg the staff never to send him anywhere again.

Back at the home, their first move was to remove the bed from his room altogether and lay the mattress directly on the floor. If he tried to get up in the night, his alarm would go off, but at least he would not have too dramatic a fall.

Meanwhile, the promised follow-on physiotherapy sessions from the hospital took rather longer to introduce than anticipated. Farrow Hall kept ringing the relevant department, as did I. "Just be patient," was the gist of the reply. Eventually, I got hold of someone in the physiotherapy unit itself and explained how, on the day Norman left, I had been promised that someone from their "outside team of physios" would appear that same week.

"I'm sorry," said the girl, "but I am that team. I did have an assistant but she's off pregnant."

The nurses at Farrow Hall did what they could to help until the day came when the physiotherapist confirmed that she would be arriving that very morning. (The visit turned out to be a disaster in that Norman was asleep and the girl said she would come back another day.) Suzi and I were sticking to our plan to go round at two o'clock but, at around one thirty, we had a phone call from Connie to say that when Norman was taken to his room for a change of shirt, he had what they termed "a funny turn". It was a TIA or minor stroke which left him momentarily unconscious.

Connie told us that he would probably sleep off the ill effects, though the chances were that he might be more muddled than he was before. She also passed on the slightly better news that the doctor was not unduly worried about Norman's condition because he had started to speak when examined. By the time Suzi and I arrived, it was as if nothing had happened.

Norman slept well that night but at lunch time the following day I had another call. Norman had had a proper stroke, one in which he had been out to the world for six or seven minutes. When he came round, his face was drooping on the right side.

I hurried round to Farrow Hall where he was sitting in the lounge and looking terrible. None of the above, though, had stopped what had become an incessant urge to get up and to walk, only now the attempts were more furious than ever. That I kept encouraging him to sit down made him still worse.

There was a new lady who had arrived in the lounge – I think she must have belonged upstairs – who was staring at the goings-on. She watched Norman's desperate efforts to stand, and she watched my desperate efforts to get him to do the opposite. Before too long, she gave her opinion.

"That woman," she said of me to a passing carer, "is perfectly able-bodied, so why isn't she helping him to get up? She threw me a look to suggest that my cruelty knew no bounds.

I had become well used to this side of dementia, to the way victims talk out loud where, previously, they would presumably have spoken in whispers if, indeed, they had not been good enough to keep their thoughts to themselves.

Alphonso stepped in to explain that I was helping Norman rather than the reverse, but the woman would not hear of it.

I tried to appease her myself, saying that if Norman were to get up, he would almost certainly fall and ruin all the good work that a surgeon had done on his hip. She looked at me disbelievingly and pulled a face.

Tori joined me while I waited for the doctor to arrive and the two of us noticed that whenever there was a pause in the up-and-down routine, Norman was breathing heavily and holding on to the right side of his head. The hostility had subsided and he confided, in the old-fashioned vernacular, "I feel queer."

It was the only sentence he had uttered and there was an unexpected flash of warmth in the way he said it.

All our married life, whenever he or anyone else was suffering in any way, he would refuse to believe it was of any consequence. (Most members of his family were no different.) For an example which was 'all Norman', there was that day when I had gone down with gastric flu when he needed me to find some ancient newspaper article in the cellar. Finally, his patience ran out. Some hammering at the bathroom door was followed by a terse, "Haven't you finished being sick, yet?"

There was another glorious example in July of 1991 when our son, Logan, was involved in a nasty climbing accident in Ecuador which left him minus the middle finger of his left hand.

Norman and I were at that year's Open at Royal Birkdale when news came that Logan, who had inherited his father's love of rugby, had just come round after a long and difficult operation. It was a worrying time and when, a few phone-calls later, Norman rang the hospital, specifically to speak to Logan, his first question was not exactly the conventional, "How are you feeling?" Instead, he was desperate to learn how the injury might affect his throwing-in. Next, he expressed concern about his golf grip and what might work for the best in the circumstances, interlocking or overlapping. Logan had to tell him that such things weren't exactly at the top of his list of priorities.

When I had my four children within the space of five years, I soon gave up on mentioning that it was mighty hard work. His early responses had always included a reference to his mother, who had 13 children and apparently never complained. (Norman would often explain how he played his part by helping with the washing up on Christmas Day.)

In all the 50-odd years we had lived in the same house, the local doctors had no idea of Norman's existence until I dared to call the surgery because of what turned out to be his first bout of osteomyelitis. Norman was furious that I had done such a thing and, when a doctor appeared, he refused to see her. The doctor said she had no option but to respect his wishes and leave but, after getting the gist of our situation, she was good enough to change her mind and to go ahead with a few tests. Norman stopped complaining when she listened to his usual diagnosis about old rugby injuries playing up again.

That day in Farrow Hall when he acknowledged that he was "feeling queer" was possibly the first time that he had ever conceded that something might be wrong. The bravado and the bitterness had disappeared. His vulnerability was unmasked and so too was the bullet-proof front I had developed over the years to deal with some at least of his difficult ways.

When the doctor turned up, he confirmed that Norman had had a proper stroke and that the only way to identify what kind of stroke it was would be to go to the hospital for a scan.

"No thanks," I said, hurriedly. It was the last thing I wanted for Norman and the last thing which Norman would have wanted for himself. The doctor understood.

Patrick and Suzi came with me the next day and, when we took to pushing Norman up and down the corridors in a wheelchair to stop him from trying to walk, he said it was "bloody awful." That, from Norman, was quite a positive response and, in the weeks that followed, he did begin to pick up a bit of strength, even if the standing-up, sitting-down routines were still failing to help.

For months, I hadn't paid much attention to my work with an American digital magazine but, at this point, I wanted to put in an appearance at an end-of-season golf tournament in Dubai. I felt the need to get back in touch though, at the same time, I was well aware that five days away from home were hardly to be recommended. I discussed it with Alphonso, who insisted that Norman's condition was stable and that the trip would not make any difference to anything, especially when my sister, Miranda, was going to be around to contribute to the daily visiting. At the same time,

Alphonso suggested that a bit of sunshine might do me good.

It probably was doing me good until that moment, a mere three days after my arrival, when I slipped on a couple of white marble steps in the newly reconstructed clubhouse. The trouble was that the builders had still to add the lighting in that area and, in the half-dark, the steps did not show up as steps. The Health and Safety official doing duty at the tournament told me how he had raised concerns about this shortcoming – and not a few others – only two days earlier.

When, four days after I had set out for Dubai, I reappeared at Farrow Hall with my foot in one of those broken-bone boots, Norman's opening remark was sufficiently acerbic to confirm that he was in pretty good shape. After a quick glance at my foot, he said, "That's your fault." There were plenty of times when I was given the blame for things which had nothing to do with me but, on this occasion, he was more right than wrong and I was not about to dispute it.

Perhaps because of the short break, I noticed something different about Norman. His non-stop efforts to get up had slowed a little, with the attempts no longer the equivalent of some desperate endeavour to add a few yards to his drives at golf. If that was not necessarily a good sign, it was still a relief to see him looking more relaxed. Patrick joined us for tea and Norman tuned into what we were saying about broken bones in the family, including one of Norman's in his rugby-playing days.

A month further on and Norman was life-weary as much as anything else. He died in his sleep shortly before Christmas and, with all those attempts to stand up finally spent, he looked at peace.

Maybe, just maybe, his last dreams were devoted to what he had so proudly announced to some of his rugby friends a few weeks earlier: the news that he had just been chosen to play football for Celtic.

Chapter 22: Short Shrift from Nakita

My return trips to play the piano following Norman's death in December 2014 acted as therapy as much as anything else. I had fainted in Marks and Spencer's the week before the funeral and, in coming round – I was leaning against a stack of oranges – I expressed surprise that Norman had died. When Patrick, who was with me at the time, was unable to get hold of Suzi, he rang Michele, who came rushing up from London earlier than planned and whisked me off to the doctor. "I'm not surprised she fainted," Dr Angela McGowan told her. In retrospect, neither was I. So much had gone on for so long.

Once I was back playing that piano, Betsy came downstairs for every session, as did Belinda, the lady with the dusters. Dorothy, Alicia, Annie and Nakita were four more regulars whose familiar foot-tapping was a cheering feature of a bleak month.

You never quite knew what you were going to get from Nakita who, in fact, had been unusually charming for several weeks. But one day, when I was halfway through what was a thoroughly cheerful routine which included a couple of Beatles numbers, Nakita, who was clearly oblivious to my efforts, stood up.

"Heard it once, heard it all before," she declared. "I'm off. Do you want to come with me, Dorothy?"

Dorothy who, amid her muddles, had often shown an acute awareness of others' feelings, looked appalled.

"That's so unkind, Nakita. Why would you say that when we love it when the pianist comes and plays for us?"

"I agree," said Betsy.

Nakita repeated her new mantra.

"Heard it once, heard it all before. I'd rather watch television."

"Go and watch your own television," said Alicia.

"I'd rather watch this one if you don't mind."

"We'd rather you didn't," said Annie.

"Please, please carry on playing," implored Dorothy as Nakita stomped off, her handbag in dangerously full swing.

I tried to carry on, but her remark had been a killer. Whatever it was that had fuelled my piano-playing at Farrow Hall had evaporated. Just like that. Unlike what had happened when that lovely young opera singer, Elizabeth, had her 'Ave Maria' interrupted by Professor Perkins, this show did not go on, at least not at Farrow Hall.

Alphonso, no doubt recognising that I had come to a more sudden halt than usual, came up and said that I wasn't to take any notice of Nakita: "She doesn't mean it."

I knew that much was true and I did not blame Nakita in any way. But it brought back too many memories of how often people had said the same on days when Norman would be delivering some of his more scathing remarks. On one level, you knew he did not mean it but, for some reason, that did not make the remarks any less hurtful. Some could be laughed off, others not. You would not have wanted them to stick, but stick they did, with one which refuses to be shrugged off even now, that of the time I said I was off for a short walk and he countered with the suggestion that I should walk under a bus.

I had a friend, Pam, who lived close by and, since her mother had died of dementia about ten years before, I asked if it had been the same for her. It had.

"It took me ages to get over some of Mum's nastier comments," she began. "They were all I could think of and it was a shame when she and I had been so close. I can promise you, though, that that stage doesn't last for ever."

She was not wrong.

Quite how long it took I cannot remember but in time the better memories, like spring flowers, began to put in an appearance. I remember the first of them. Patrick had come round one evening and, as we wondered what we should have to eat, he hit on fish and chips. "You and dad used to enjoy going down to Harry Ramsden's for a fish supper," he recalled. [Harry Ramsden's was a splendid fish and chip restaurant down the coast.]

For the next few moments, I was all three of stunned, bemused and silent. I could not argue the point.

Postscript

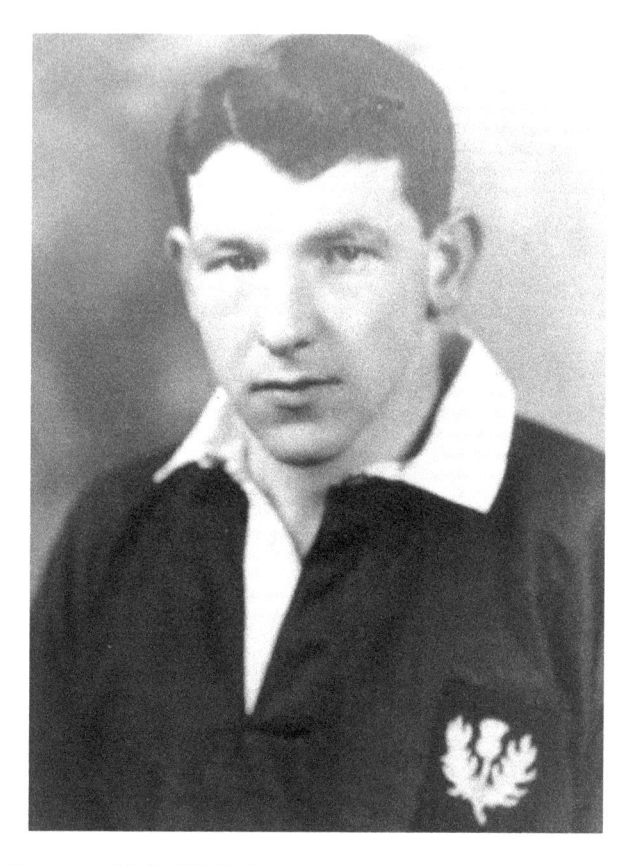

Norman Mair MBE: October 1928 – December 2014

Excerpts from Norman Mair obituaries.

Alasdair Reid:

"In the language of the sports pages, greatness is plentiful," wrote Hugh McIlvanney, one of the very few who could stand shoulder to shoulder with Norman, in response to the death of Sir Matt Busby in 1994. "The reality of sport, like that of every other area of life, is that it is desperately rare. Greatness does not gad about, reaching for people in handfuls. It settles deliberately on a blessed few."

It settled on Norman when he took his first steps in sportswriting more than half a century ago, and it stayed there until he put down his pen around 45 years later. Like the legendary football and boxing writer John Rafferty, with whom he formed a formidable partnership at *The Scotsman*, he came to journalism after spending time as a teacher and it is fair to say that something of the dominie lingered both in his bearing and his prose. Reading him was always an education.

The Merchistonian, anon:

On 3 February 1951, 22-year-old NGR Mair (42-47) boarded the team bus outside the North British Hotel and headed off down to Murrayfield to win the second of his four rugby caps. This was his home debut and was against a highly-rated Welsh XV which featured 11 British Lions.

The 81,000-strong crowd had been swelled by a selection of Norman's six sisters and five surviving brothers.

Against all the odds, Scotland prevailed by the then record margin of 19-0. It would be the highlight of NGR Mair's rugby career.

Norman was as well read as many academics and had an encyclopaedic knowledge of Shakespeare, the great poets and a wide variety of classical and contemporary texts. If, as Allan Massie, a Fellow of the Royal Society of Literature, wrote in his much-appreciated obituary, there were echoes of PG Wodehouse in Norman's writing, it was not surprising. Wodehouse's books were always more worn than the others on Norman's shelves.

Along with his sense of humour, Norman's literary background formed the foundation of any number of his anecdotes. Readers were frequently astounded at his ability to reference so wide an array of sources. The essence of his writing was beautifully captured in a book called *Stargazing*, which tells the story of lighthouse keepers working off Scotland's west coast.

The author recorded how Ross, one of the lighthouse keepers, would eagerly await the twice weekly boat from the mainland bearing vital provisions. To Ross, no provision was more vital than Norman's latest columns in *The Scotsman*.

Alan Pattullo: *The Scotsman*:

Jim Telfer, who played for Scotland and the Lions and was head coach to the British and Irish Lions on their tour of New Zealand in 1983, described Mair as the written word's equivalent to Bill McLaren, who was described as the "voice of rugby" when the much-loved commentator passed away four years ago.

"Norman is a great loss," said Telfer. "Bill McLaren and Norman are of the old generation – you don't get them very often. He was a friend as well as a journalist. He used to come into my office at Murrayfield just for a blether and he always had something new to tell you even though he was 70 years old by then. He was always ahead of the game, never mind up with it."

Martin Dempster, *The Scotsman*:

According to Allan Massie, Norman Mair had "no equals in Scottish rugby writing". In the eyes of Stephen Jones (*Sunday Times*), he will "always remain my favourite rugby writer of all time". Praise indeed from admired figures in the oval ball game.

Instant tributes may have been less forthcoming from what could probably be described as his "second sport" but, nonetheless, golf has also been saddened by the death at 86 of one of its iconic writers.

Having joined the Association of Golf Writers 1966, Norman George Robertson Mair, a quintessential Edinburgh man, was one of the Association's longest-standing members. He was held in the same regard as Bernard Darwin and Peter Dobereiner, which tells you instantly that he was blessed with a special talent.

Stephen Jones, *Sunday Times*:

Terribly sad at the passing of Norman Mair, who will always remain my favourite rugby writer of all time. Beautiful essayist and gracious man.

Lewine Mair

Lewine Mair was the first woman to be signed on as a sports' correspondent for a national daily paper. She was with the *Daily Telegraph* for 18 years, six of them covering sport in general and the remaining 12 as the paper's golf correspondent. She has also written for *The Times* and, today, is a regular contributor to the American digital magazine, *Global Golf Post*.

She has interviewed such as Tiger Woods, Donald Trump and Rod Laver along the way, while she is also the author of *Carefree Golf*, the story of Dame Laura Davies, and *The Real Monty*, which covers Colin Montgomerie's life and golf. *Tapping Feet, a Doubletake on Care Homes and Dementia*, is her first book on a different theme.

A winner of the Rolex award for sportswriting, Mair has been short-listed three times for the British Sportswriter of the Year awards.

Lightning Source UK Ltd.
Milton Keynes UK
UKHW022228140223
416982UK00012B/760